WHEN BREASTFEEDING SUCKS

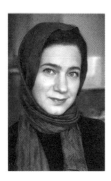

About the author

Zainab Yate BSc, MSc (Medical Ethics & Law, Imperial College London) is an independent researcher and campaigner, and published the first study looking at breastfeeding/nursing aversion and agitation in 2017.

She has been a breastfeeding peer supporter with the NHS for a number of years and is author of the only resource site for mothers and healthcare practitioners on aversion (www.breastfeedingaversion.com), where she researches and writes about aversion and why it arises. She has helped thousands of women when breastfeeding triggers negative emotions through her free structured support course and peer to peer support group online.

Her working background is in public health and commissioning within the NHS and she is currently vice-chair and named qualitative lead of the North London Research Ethics Committee, with the Health Research Authority in the UK (HRA). She is also a member of the Kings College London Research Ethics, Governance Policy & Integrity Committee (KCL). In both roles she is a breastfeeding advocate and infant feeding research ethics expert for the committees.

WHEN
BREASTFEEDING
SUCKS

What you need to know about
nursing aversion and agitation

Zainab Yate

To my husband. The development of this book and the possibility to write it came about due to your consistent insight and support.

To the mothers struggling with aversion, who have braced the possible onslaught of judgement, and openly shared their struggles with breastfeeding with me, both online and off.

When Breastfeeding Sucks:
What you need to know about nursing aversion and agitation

First published in the UK by Pinter & Martin Ltd 2020

Copyright © Zainab Yate 2020

ISBN 978-1-78066-685-3

Also available as an ebook

The right of Zainab Yate to be identified as the author of this work has been asserted by her in accordance with the Copyright, Designs and Patent Act of 1988

Edited by Susan Last
Index by Helen Bilton
Proofread by Tamsin English

British Library Cataloguing-in-Publication Data

A catalogue record for this book is available from the British Library

Printed in the EU by Hussar

This book has been printed on paper that is sourced and harvested from sustainable forests and is FSC accredited

Pinter & Martin Ltd
6 Effra Parade
London SW2 1PS

pinterandmartin.com

Contents

Introduction

It first happened when my daughter was five months old, it was the middle of the night and I had only just managed to get to sleep myself after the last feed when she woke again for another feed. I had to sit up, get the pillows in place and get her on in seconds – otherwise she would start screaming. I remember feeling a strange creepy crawly feeling under my skin, and then I was so angry when she latched. I was feeding at night and I was so tired, so so tired: but this feeling was new, and it scared me. When was this going to get better, I used to think? Everyone kept saying it would, but it seemed to be getting worse. I felt trapped in that room, tied to the bed, held hostage because I made milk. She refused to take a bottle, I tried to express milk and my husband would hold her to offer it but she would just squirm and turn her face, what could we do? She spat dummies out within seconds, despite repeated attempts to offer them. It was only me [that could offer milk and comfort] and I started to dread feeding because I got so angry. I wasn't in pain any more – sure it wasn't a great feeling to feed, and I had to refrain from unlatching her, but not toe-curling pain. It got to the point where I was biting down on my hand while she fed – just to get through the feed. I felt like a monster when she was on, it was scary. And when she stopped feeding it would go away, but I just felt so guilty. I mean what kind of mother feels like that when she is feeding her baby? Outside, it was like silent suffocation, pretending that I loved breastfeeding like everyone else. It was only when

I found an article online about breastfeeding aversion and agitation I realised it was a thing. As I read it I just cried and cried. I felt like it was describing exactly what I was going through, like they were my exact words, my story, my feelings, my despair at the situation, and what I felt every day. I can't describe to you the relief I felt, knowing that it wasn't only me.
Felicity, London

'I want to rip my breasts off'

In her critically acclaimed book *Mothers: An Essay on Love and Cruelty*, Jacqueline Rose argues that mothers are punished just for being mothers while being instructed to 'love without reserve'. Rose cites deluded expectations of motherhood and states that a mother's hate in its intensity matches her love.[*] Proportionality and disproportionality are underlying themes discussed in her book. This book too covers our expectations as mothers, and considers what are normal responses in the situation of a mother who experiences difficulties and challenges when breastfeeding – and questions, without reserve, what could cause them and why. I deconstruct what a proportional emotional response is when breastfeeding becomes a difficult situation and a mother experiences breastfeeding as triggering negative emotions, otherwise known as breastfeeding aversion and agitation – or aversion for short. If you have not heard of aversion, it can take a little time to adjust to the raw, frank and honest descriptions of breastfeeding with it that some mothers have.

Does the statement 'I want to rip my breasts off' alarm you? If it does, I can probably wager you haven't experienced severe aversion. If you had, you would be shaking your head from side to side, saying 'nope' out loud, and, with a heavy heart, thinking of a time – perhaps not long ago – when you felt like you wanted to do just that to your own breasts. You had just had enough of breastfeeding, perhaps of mothering in general: you didn't want to be the source of milk, the *only*

---

[*]   Rose, J. (2018). *Mothers: An Essay on Love and Cruelty* (Main edition). London: Faber & Faber, p97

source of milk, you didn't want to be woken up 15 times last night, or punched, scratched, stroked, or even touched – you wanted to have your body *as your own*. Breastfeeding was becoming tiresome. Did you not love breastfeeding anymore? You positively hated it. And hate, we are not often told, can exist in and among love.

Naomi Stadlen wrote about love and hate being coexisting forces in her book *What Mothers Do.*[*] Reading it opened my mind to a broader, more flexible way of thinking about who we are as mothers and the varying ways of love. How we love, how much we love, and how some of us cannot love or feel unable to love due to our circumstances or our upbringing. While researching this book, I looked into how societal ideas of love and motherhood have changed over time. Did you know that in the 15th century motherhood didn't carry expectations of emotions and sentiments like it does now with the notion of 'motherly love'? It was only later, in the 18th century, that the feelings, behaviours and responsibilities of mothers were taken very seriously. Women were increasingly expected to feel a close bond with their children, and their maternal qualities were judged and evaluated by this bond.[**] In our current age of scientific knowledge about neuroscience and the role of hormones in biology, we recognise that having secure attachment is important for humans to thrive. Yet, we as mothers have to recognise that our own ideas about motherhood are not determined by biology alone, but also by society.

A mother's love is epitomised as the purest, most natural love, placed on a high pedestal, and in the 19th century it started to be idealised in literature. This propagated the idea that there is something uniquely special and innate about a mother's love. A natural consequence of this over the centuries has been the erasure of a mother's hate, meaning that mothers have been disallowed to feel certain things because they would be judged, silenced or condemned. It is now a failing

---

[*]   Stadlen, Naomi. (2007). *What mothers do, especially when it looks like nothing.* New York: Jeremy P. Tarcher/Penguin.
[**] Hays, S. (1998). *The Cultural Contradictions of Motherhood.* Yale University Press.

on a mother's part if she does not fit into the picturesque, quintessential idea of an all-giving mother, who loves her child and sacrifices all for them. There is nothing wrong with this kind of pseudo-martyrdom, as it is biologically normal and indeed essential to do this in the newborn period, but what about afterwards? What about the fact that it is not possible to 'give your all' as a mother in 21st-century life? To be a wholesome, perfect mother while working, or managing other children and conflicting responsibilities without something giving way, or without some trade-off, is impossible. Whether it is your mental health, your bodily health, your financial health, your family's health, or your children's health, you will always drop a ball at some point in this juggling act. Maybe once a day, maybe all day. According to Hays, getting it right has always been out of reach for mothers, keeping us constantly striving and never quite getting there.[*] We will 'fail', and according to Rose, failing is normal and expected. What isn't normal and expected is how society views mothers, and how it responds to their suffering. After reading Rose's essay, I began to wonder about aversion in the breastfeeding journey. How many mothers simply do not know that you can experience negative emotions when breastfeeding? Hating breastfeeding is so hidden that some mothers think they are the only ones that feel that way. I wondered, isn't the erasure of hate worse than the hate itself? I believe we set mothers up for further failure when we don't talk about the challenges of negative emotions when breastfeeding, in the reality of this lived 21st-century motherhood. I wondered what the extent of this problem was, and so I began to research it.

In an exploratory study I conducted in 2017 to describe the phenomenon, I found that women all over the world are experiencing aversion – which is when breastfeeding triggers particular 'negative' emotions like anger and agitation and intrusive thoughts, often with an overwhelming urge to de-latch a suckling baby or child.[**] I also found that aversion is

---

[*] Hays, S. (1998). *The Cultural Contradictions of Motherhood.* Yale University Press.

[**] Yate, Z. (2017). A qualitative study on negative emotions triggered by breastfeeding; Describing the phenomenon of breastfeeding/nursing

not only experienced if you are pregnant and breastfeeding, or tandem breastfeeding two children, but also if you are breastfeeding only one infant, even a newborn, and are not pregnant. Seemingly, *any* breastfeeding woman can experience aversion. In online support groups and through my resource site, some women have reported that they experience the same negative feelings of aversion when expressing or pumping milk from their breasts. The peer reviewed study, which was included in a systematic review and quality assessed using the Critical Appraisal Skills Programme (CASP) checklist, contributes to the 'hidden realities' of infant feeding.*

Even though there are few pieces of published academic or clinical literature on aversion, and there is relatively little known in a medical sense about *why* breastfeeding causes negative emotions in some mothers, there is more than enough to indicate the existence of the phenomenon. There are too many women with too many questions that remain unanswered about aversion, who wonder who they are as mothers when they experience aversion. This is because experiencing aversion can disrupt the emotional, physical and psychological balance that offering the breast can ordinarily achieve, which can be devastating for mothers and nurslings, and for family life in general. This book is a rather lengthy attempt to explain aversion, both for the mothers who experience it and for the healthcare practitioners or lactation specialists who are supporting mothers though it.

Who am I, as a mother?

Firstly, if you are breastfeeding, the chances are you *want* to do it, because, let's face it, getting a milk supply established is no mean feat. Secondly, it is also likely that you know all about the health, social, and mental benefits that breastfeeding

aversion and agitation in breastfeeding mothers. *Iranian Journal of Nursing and Midwifery Research, 22*(6), 449.

* Dattilo, A. M., Carvalho, R. S., Feferbaum, R., Forsyth, S., & Zhao, A. (2020a). Hidden Realities of Infant Feeding: Systematic Review of Qualitative Findings from Parents. Behavioral Sciences, 10(5), 83. doi. org/10.3390/bs10050083

offers your child, and you as a lactating mother. Unless you've been hiding under a proverbial rock, you will have had this information thrust at you at every opportunity since you started carrying your little pea in your belly. Thirdly, it goes without saying that you love your nursling in your way ('nurslings' if you are a superwoman goddess tandem feeder or feeder of multiples). So given these three things, and the fact that you as a rational adult and mother have autonomously decided to breastfeed, *why* then are you starting to hate breastfeeding, getting angry, and having this urge to de-latch your nursling and deny them milk when they want or need it? There is no simple answer, and that is why there is a whole book dedicated to answering this question.

Whether you are a first-time mother or a boobie veteran, aversion can strike at any point in a breastfeeding journey. It's much more serious than feeling tetchy a few times while breastfeeding. Having aversion can mean battling against what your body and part of your mind is telling you to do ('get this kid off me'), and it can create a constant emotional burden that includes guilt and shame about feeling the way you do when you feed. Even though mothers can struggle with aversion once or occasionally, it is very common to experience it monthly. Some mothers experience it daily, and others at every single feed. For many, aversion rears its ugly head when you least expect it, and often it doesn't just 'go away'.

This book is the result of my endeavour to try to understand aversion for the better part of a decade, from the lectures I have given, from listening to and supporting mothers, from my structured support course online and from my own reading and personal deliberation. I found that the courses I took, the support I gave to mothers, and literature in the area of infant feeding and breastfeeding did not help answer questions about who I was as a mother who experienced aversion, let alone what aversion itself was and why I was experiencing it. In fact, the more I became involved in the breastfeeding world, the less I knew who I was as a breastfeeding mother. I didn't fit into the typical model of a happily-in-love breastfeeding mother and baby couple or 'dyad'. And although I read hundreds of articles and books, the negative feelings that breastfeeding can trigger were rarely referred to, let alone addressed. I had to look deeper, read between the lines and make links with other fields of research in order to arrive at answers.

Despite having a difficult breastfeeding journey, and experiencing severe aversion, I wanted to continue to breastfeed, and I wanted to help other mothers to breastfeed. However, it was really difficult to reconcile this desire to continue breastfeeding with the fact that I really hated breastfeeding. Sure, I *wanted* to love it, and there were perhaps a handful of moments over the four years I was breastfeeding when I did (maybe) *like* it, and there were definitely a few occasions when I was infinitely grateful that I was *able* to breastfeed. But on the whole it was a long, difficult, painful, heart-wrenching, heart-breaking, emotionally burdening, body-changing, character-testing experience – which I personally think made my relationship with my children worse, contrary to what breastfeeding is normatively understood to do. It was difficult to talk openly about aversion years ago: there was no one in my personal or professional life, nor in my breastfeeding groups and online circles, who seemed to experience it. No one spoke frankly about despising breastfeeding *while* doing it.

So for a long time it was difficult to accept the personal experience of aversion in myself as a breastfeeding mother. Looking back, it was a little odd to think that I was continuing an activity I had rationally concluded that I hated, which was clearly having a negative impact on my mental health and my overall home-life balance. I think that's why I started to work on finding the words to explain what aversion was – and now, thanks to hundreds of other women who experienced the same as me and were brave enough to open up, those words are published in an open source article.

Once I realised that other women experienced aversion, and that they too often thought it was 'only me', I began work on social media to raise awareness in the breastfeeding community so that others knew they were not alone. The nature of all (popular) social media posts is to present a good life, one that is desirable, even enviable. For us as mothers, presumably, it is to portray mothering with effortlessness and grace, breastfeeding with smiles and love. In short, being 'happy' as a mother. But behind the elegant photography and the wise words posted, we don't actually know how many of the posts are from mothers that *have* got it all together, and I think that's the point. Even though social media in some ways celebrated and normalised breastfeeding, in the end we all hide behind smiles. I realised that I had to celebrate breastfeeding in all its glory, but also show its ugly side. Using the hashtags #aversionsucks and #touchedout really opened up space for honest stories of struggle from women who experienced aversion, alongside those who didn't, which is exactly where I wanted it to be to normalise negative feelings when breastfeeding and connect with the mothers who struggled. Only when I started this did I begin to see the real desperation that affected mothers who had aversion and didn't know why, and couldn't get rid of it.

Next I started researching aversion more seriously, to understand why it happens, and what we could do about it. From a starting point of hopelessness and despair (aversion never left me once it hit, and I had to reluctantly wean both my children because of it), I found some insights that I knew could help women, and I am hopeful that it may be possible to address aversion in some dyads.

Before we get into my theory on what aversion is, and what can help, I want to set the scene. I cannot assume that everyone understands the importance of breastfeeding in mothering, nor the importance of breastmilk itself for some mothers (and, of course, their nurslings). To this end, I want to highlight two important concepts that lay the foundations for understanding breastfeeding as an activity in a wider context of mothering, and why many women continue to breastfeed despite experiencing a phenomenon that urges them to de-latch their nursling or even stop breastfeeding altogether. These concepts, I believe, really help us understand why some mothers may experience aversion in the first place. The first is 'skinship', and the second 'nurture'. The former is taken from Japanese culture, the latter from the Arabic language using an analysis of linked root words.

PART I

The Love and
The Hate

1

Touch and 'Skinship'

Touch that builds relationships, touch that breaks it

The notion that physical closeness and skin contact can create a kind of intimate bond is something instinctively known to humans, and has been discussed extensively in academic and cultural literature. Most parents know the importance of skin-to-skin, and that breastfeeding is inextricably bound to this repeated physical closeness. Yet, when experiencing aversion, the notion that this repeated contact with skin builds a loving and secure relationship is brought into question. Especially when we consider the emotions aversion triggers of anger or agitation, intrusive thoughts and the 'urge to de-latch' and 'run away' or 'push the nursling off'. Although many can suppress this urge, breastfeeding with aversion can mean prematurely ending a breastfeeding session because of these emotions and thoughts – with both parties in tears. This seems to be the exact *opposite* of what closeness, skin contact and breastfeeding is supposed to bring.

With what many of us consider loving mothering to be – including responsive parenting and night-time care – we may find ourselves as mothers spending much of our time holding, feeding, and touching our babies, infants or children, often for hours each day, regardless of their age. While the immediate dependency of a newborn for survival is demonstrably time-consuming, when we consider teething, illness, family disruption and a whole array of other factors, mothering responsively is *always* time consuming in the early years and doesn't ever actually stop. To understand these daily (and nightly) activities with the intimate nature of the breastfeeding relationship and how this relationship is compromised when aversion strikes we turn now to look at the concept of *skinship*.

Skinship is actually originally an English word, but is now considered to come from the Japanese, and is a mix of two words or a 'portmanteau' of the English words 'skin' and 'friendship'. It uniquely describes an interaction through skin contact that builds love or closeness, and was initially, and historically, used to convey touch between a mother and child. Skinship is a widespread, deeply rooted concept in traditional and modern-day Japanese culture, although it now more commonly refers to intimate touching in romantic relationships. Regardless of its application to a relationship, touch and touchability are a key theme of the Japanese concept of skinship. And skinship can help us understand the importance of touch for mothers and how this relates to aversion.

The meaning of touch

To be human is to feel things, to touch and be touched. Touch is a form of social glue as it binds sexual partners into lifetime partners, siblings in families and even individuals in a work team. Different forms of celebratory touch in various sports have been shown to affect game outcomes for the better. To be human is also to be emotional: touch or even a sense of touch will arouse different emotions and is intrinsically emotional. There is a deep connection between emotion and the sense of touch. We know severe touch deprivation causes neuropsychiatric problems, including cognitive delays and attachment disorders, stunted growth, gastrointestinal problems and overall negative effects on the immune system. The well-known story of babies and children in Romanian orphanages that were fed, but not ever held, taught the world that touch is a biological condition necessary for human development, and for human existence itself. The children in the orphanages often did not survive long, and those that did suffered lifelong effects from neglect. Psychologist Harlow's famous experiments on rhesus monkeys had also suggested what we now know: frequent touch is needed in the first two years of life, or problems from a lack of touch will persist for the rest of life, regardless of whether touch interventions occur afterwards. Touch, or touchability, continues as a main and basic defining characteristic of all familial relations, of course with the proviso that touch is from those you trust or are close to. And this touchability as the foundation of the basis of skinship is premised on closeness and (consensual) intimacy.

The beginning of this touch-intimacy for a mother and nursling will start at birth, ideally with the physical practice of skin-to-skin to allow the baby to root for the breast, to regulate their heartbeat, their temperature, and to calm them after the unsettling journey of birth. The benefits of skin-to-skin are not disputed, and much research has been put into clinical practice all over the world to ensure that mothers and babies are able to have skin-to-skin – ideally from the very first minute, but if not then during the first 'golden hour' of life outside the womb, regardless of delivery route. Breastfeeding itself necessarily results in skin-to-skin contact due to spatial proximity, and is attributed to promoting and solidifying bonds over time. From the lips, mouth and cheek as a minimum, there is reciprocal skin contact for the baby and the mother, and the boundaries between the two of them are blurred, as you cannot really tell where the mother's body ends and the nursling's begins.* It is generally understood that you cannot 'touch' one way, because touch is necessarily a two-way thing, as both persons will experience sensations of touch. A sort of reversibility.** Breastfeeding, and therefore touch, to establish supply and to adequately nourish a newborn baby's growth, happens very regularly: at least every 2–3 hours in the early weeks and months.

Alongside this outward physical contact, there is a deeper, more ephemeral bond which Tahhan calls 'touching at depth'

---

*   Tahhan, D. A. (2014). *The Japanese Family: Touch, Intimacy and Feeling*. Routledge, (Claudels 1972, p195)

**   Ibid, p167

in her book on the Japanese family that looks at bonding through intimate spaces. She outlines a sort of relational understanding of touch that is not located in a particular part of the body.[*] That this kind of special 'touch' grows with physical proximity and touchability is not often spoken about or celebrated, because of recent decades of incorrect advice to ignore babies' needs as they were considered 'manipulative'. This advice has led to responsiveness being frowned upon, and age-old bed-sharing practices and night-time care to be shunned by society in many Western countries.

'Anshin' is the Japanese word that describes what comes with shared sleep ('soine'), or bed-sharing, which is a practice that is woven through the fabric of family life in many parts of the world. The state of anshin is the 'feeling of contentment and relief' or 'peace of the heart', and the Japanese consider that bed-sharing and breastfeeding facilitate this anshin for parents and children: it benefits the whole family. The intimacy of anshin that arises with the particular nature of a relationship formed with skinship is at the very foundation of familial relations and family connection, second only to sharing of blood and DNA. Perhaps because of this, anshin is something that we assume will be as beautiful and natural as breastfeeding or mothering itself. And so long as the boundary-less connection of positive touch exists, and feelings of contentment and security are felt by mother and nursling, anshin can be a beautiful and natural development of the all-encompassing space which the breastfeeding relationship can take up. When breastfeeding is working, and is easy for a mother, it can be relaxing in a deep way, which can promote skinship and anshin. But when breastfeeding is painful, or uncomfortable, or becomes difficult for a mother to sustain, it will not promote this contented state. And many mothers do not realise there are challenging parts to creating anshin through skinship – with personal, physical and emotional obstacles to overcome when breastfeeding responsively during the day, and co-sleeping or bed-sharing at night as so many breastfeeding mothers do.

---

[*]   Ibid, foreword, xvii.

When touch is a trigger

Intimate touch is often assumed to be consensual when we think of a mother and nursling, and a mother's consent to be touched is presumed if a baby is the other party in the interaction. This makes sense as babies are not autonomous persons, they cannot make rational decisions and are wholly dependent on their mother or primary caregiver for their survival. They are not required to gain consent to touch because they cannot. Yet some women have negative feelings that can arise from being touched when they do not want to be, or in a way they do not want to be. I have seen this less often in the newborn period, although it does occur, but certainly touch becomes an issue as mothers breastfeed into toddlerhood and breastfeed older children. There are aspects of bodily autonomy, and feelings of not consenting to being touched, which are not generally addressed in breastfeeding mothers, because consent is generally understood in an adult-to-adult capacity and not within a concept of maternal autonomy.

> *I just don't feel like I have any power over my body, it's like I don't really own it anymore as the milk is theirs, and when they clamber on me and reach into my top to nurse I can't say no as they need to feed.* Kathryn, Wendover

We think of touch as a unified sensation, but there are many different kinds of nerve endings that specialise in the transfer of certain kinds of information. For example, merkel endings are dense in sensitive parts of the body, like the tongue, the fingertip and the cornea.[*] We have differing nerve endings for heat, cold, vibration, pressure and pain, and the density of each of these in a part of the skin gives rise to different personal experiences. So when looking at the importance of touch we must not assume that all touch is 'good', or even that all touch is important, but that specific facets of touch

---

[*]   Halata, Z., Grim, M., & Baumann, K. I. (2010). Current understanding of Merkel cells, touch reception and the skin. *Expert Review of Dermatology*, 5(1), 109–116.

profoundly affect our human experience. And as we have different levels of sensory preferences and tolerance, perhaps due to our genetic makeup, touch can be uncomfortable or painful for some mothers but not for others. And touch is important when we look at aversion, because many argue that there are no sensations without emotions. In many ways we are just sensory-emotional processing machines, and all our nerve endings provide us with the information to process. All the streams of information from the merkel endings come to the spinal cord and then the brain. They are distributed into two different systems. The first is the somatosensory cortex. This registers where in the body you are being touched and how intensely. The second is the posterior insular, which is what gives different kinds of touch their emotional frequency or 'tone'.[*] Many of us think that certain sensations have an emotional tone, for example that being pinched or hit will cause a negative response, but it is actually only because these two systems are active at the same time that we get this kind of negative response. In short, not everyone will experience the same emotions with the same external stimuli.

Mothers with aversion speak about what triggers their negative emotions, including variations of different kinds of touch, movement or sensations and consequently the subsequent feelings that are not pleasurable and not welcome. Common triggers are nipple tweaking or twiddling, scratching, pinching, and even gentle stroking by their nursling. Sensitive parts of the body like the nipple can be culprit areas, but triggers are very individualised and can also be in other areas of the body depending on the kinds of touch. Triggers can also be exacerbated in certain situations, such as at night or in response to individual mothers' external life pressures and expectations. On a very basic level, having to breastfeed when you do not want to, or when you feel you ought to be doing something more pressing, can exacerbate triggers – and so in turn cause aversion. And, as you can imagine, there can be an array of other reasons mothers may

---

[*]   Linden, D. J. (2016). *Touch: The Science of the Hand, Heart, and Mind* (Reprint edition). Penguin Books.

have to be triggered – whether it is painful to breastfeed, they are bursting for the loo, or they have to submit their thesis next week. We will explore these reasons and confounding tensions in more detail throughout the book, and I will show how it is normal to feel aversion as a manifestation of tension that pulls you in opposite directions, but how *persistent* aversion is a sign that something is not quite right. If changes or adjustments are not made, the negative feelings of anger or agitation that arise due to breastfeeding with certain kinds of touch can actually start to bring about an emotional separation between the mother and infant. It can lead to a physical separation because of de-latching or the ultimate need to wean the child off the breast. This is because aversion can create momentary feelings of uncertainty in the mother about her love for the nursling and her ability to mother, and also an uneasiness or incompleteness due to the fact that the physical form of intimacy no longer exists in the way it 'ought to'. By this I mean it does not have the calm, loving effect that breastfeeding and skin contact with touch normally does. The reason for this may be in part because of oxytocin. Aside from its involvement in the milk let-down reflex, oxytocin is also released in response to low intensity stimulation of the skin – during touch – and positive interactions between people.* Bluntly, it seems that the 'oxytocin effect' that breastfeeding is so well known for is not working for mothers with aversion. Is this purely because of a biological pathway that is not working properly? I wouldn't think so. As we are such complex beings, there will be an array of factors that may contribute to what seems to be inhibited oxytocin. Contrary to the Cartesian assumption that the mind and body are separate, for a hug, kiss or human touch to be meaningful at all, more than just the physical body is needed, for both parties. Skinship describes bonding through touch, but there is an implicit assumption in the concept that it is touch that improves the relationship, not touch that doesn't, or seems to make it worse. Whether touch

---

*   Uvnäs-Moberg, K., Handlin, L., & Petersson, M. (2014a). Self-sooth-
      ing behaviors with particular reference to oxytocin release induced by
      non-noxious sensory stimulation. *Frontiers in Psychology*, 5, 1529.

is experienced in a positive way that builds a relationship, or a negative way that does not, is dependent on many interlinked and layered factors that we will explore throughout this book.

The concept of skinship is essential to one of the main themes of this book: the embodied experience and emotions of connection and disconnect in the intimate spaces of breastfeeding. Intimate touch between the mother and baby, which is argued to be one main form of skinship by Tahaan, is facilitated and often enhanced by breastfeeding, but this is not the case for every breastfeeding mother and nursling. And it is not the case for mothers who experience aversion in any kind of lasting or severe way. When aversion strikes, and especially if it doesn't just 'go away', it compromises the bond that can be formed and strengthened though skinship. This is because we are hardwired to pay attention to sensations that originate from the outside world, so if touch becomes uncomfortable or is not wanted, we cannot simply ignore it in the way that we can when we suppress sensations that originate from us.* And although we have been told that we can reliably take information from the outside world and make completely rational and non-emotional decisions based on this information, our senses simply do not give us the most accurate representation of the outside world. By design, our senses actually mess with the data we receive to emphasise certain bits of information and downplay others. And this happens before you are even aware of it, because by the time you are aware of the external information, the data that has been collected has already been synthesised with your emotional state, your genetic expectations from your DNA, your personal expectations and your own experiences that you have accrued through life.** Your brain will then serve them all to you as 'real'. Thus, for example, if a mother who is a survivor of previous sexual abuse is woken at night by her nursling clambering on her to breastfeed, she may find it very difficult to separate this experience of touch from her past,

---

* We automatically suppress sensations that come from inside us, which is why it is hard to tickle yourself.

** Linden, D. J. (2016). *Touch: The Science of the Hand, Heart, and Mind* (Reprint edition). Penguin Books.

more traumatic and invasive incidences of touch.

This chapter shows us that skinship is inextricably linked to breastfeeding and that touch is linked to emotion. We are one step closer to understanding how breastfeeding can trigger negative emotions. But before we go any further we have to understand why breastfeeding is important to us as mothers, and why we would continue to breastfeed despite having negative emotions when our nurslings are latched. To do this we can begin by looking at how motherhood has changed over the centuries, and how breastfeeding and nurture are intertwined as can be seen in Figure 1.

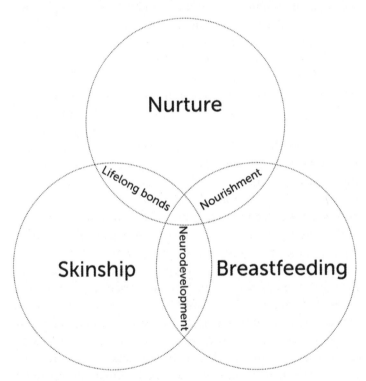

Figure 1: Mothering in Practice – How Breastfeeding, Nurture and Touch are Intertwined

2

Nursing and Nurture

Stories about families and motherhood now emerging thanks to social media are very different to mainstream ideals of motherhood. Ideals that many mothers feel are completely impossible to obtain. Having well-behaved children, a clean and orderly home, being happy and looking well-groomed while also having to work is impossible for many women, and becomes even more so with each addition to the family. Yet mothers are both expected to achieve the impossible and expect themselves to do so, because of the era they were born into, with the dominant 20th and 21st-century narratives of motherhood. I will explain. If we turn to centuries past, the main narratives of motherhood were not as they are now, and in fact changed only recently in human history. After the 19th century, rising living standards dramatically changed a mother's role, freeing up time to concentrate on her children's development. This allowed society to create a new narrative in which 'good mothers' were those who sacrificed everything in order to raise their children, and 'bad mothers' were an exception to the rule, an aberration. Twentieth-century notions of motherhood then took on psychological connotations with the rise of attachment theory. Proponents argued that the close attachment required for successful human development necessitated secure attachment with one significant figure: usually the mother. Today, in the 21st century, the focus is not specifically on mothers, but parental relationships, which are measured in reference to scientific knowledge of child development and psychology. It is purported that a child's secure attachment and interaction with a primary caregiver shapes that child's health and economic outcomes. Good attachment in the early years also teaches children that they are worthy of love, and that the world is safe. But while we progress with movements championing women's freedom and equality of rights, it is still mothers that have the main parental responsibility as primary caregivers. This is a significant role and a lifelong commitment, which we apparently ought to fulfil alongside meaningful careers. Mothers alone have this time-sensitive opportunity for the apparently unique attachment that they can have with their child in the first few formative years of life. And with milk-sharing practices and wet nursing no longer common, there is no option to 'offload' arguably the most intensive period of caring for a child if you are breastfeeding. This is perhaps one reason why mothers turn to formula feeding: if breastfeeding is not living up to the ideal we have been inculcated with, and is taking a lot more time and energy than expected, it is understandable that women seek to reduce their load. Further, the only offers of respite mothers get, both mentally and physically, are to have others feed the baby. Ideas of motherhood have changed remarkably over the years, and the notions of maternal atonement and maternal love are not as natural, nor as common, as we are led to believe. Unless we spend time researching mothers and motherhood in history, we would not know that our current society has its own version of motherhood, and others do not.

While mothers are actively pressured to 'bounce back', and to be more and do more than just mothering, including returning to work, wider society hasn't moved away from expecting mothers to carry the largest part of the childcare. To labour this point, I am saying that as a mother, which is a full-time job, you are expected to take another. And to add insult to injury, home life is no longer considered work. So it is not considered worthy of payment, having concessions for, or needing respite from. But home life was always work life, although perhaps less skilled. The two were often interlinked. Farming households, for example, brought up children inside the home as they ran the farm outside the home. They would give children food, keep them clean and teach them how to farm: looking after their future investment for the continuation of the farm. This was motherhood, raising children as you would raise farm animals, with the purpose of livelihood from both. It was only in the 18th century that this narrative began to change, because it was no longer about simply keeping children alive: it became about nurturing. The childrearing culture was born. This shift is referred to by some as the 'cult of maternity', and was represented in fiction and poetry, and prescriptive societal and medical advice, with an increase in maternal and paediatric medical intervention. The baby or child became too important to be left with paid carers, as had been commonly practised in many cultures in centuries gone by. And with this change, motherhood changed from a biological state to a more moral one, in which the mother's personal and social role had the primary concern of the well-being of her child. A devoted mother, by extension of fulfilling this primary concern, would therefore feel that all her needs were met and rewarded by her child's growth, development and activity. This was thought to be enough to give mothers self-satisfaction, and for them to be happy: maternal devotion was the truest form of love. Popular works in literature and poetry, notably *Advice to Mothers* by the famous physician and author William Buchan, and poems like 'A Mother's Love', use words like 'noble', 'pure' and 'tender' to describe mothers' love. The idealisation of motherhood is still prevalent in our current society. However, although we now have more women in the workforce, we still have policies embedded into our lives that actively prevent us from achieving the ideal of being an all-giving, all-loving mother: for example, the fact that in the United States many mothers must return to work after only six weeks, due to a lack of paid maternity leave. Mothers can feel a deep sense of shame and guilt if they don't live up to this image of motherhood, and often feel that they have failed, especially if they mother through breastfeeding. Some even feel that, because of this failure, they have missed their chance to do right by their children. We see this despair – at the thought of having irreversibly harmed their nurslings – manifest itself when mothers experience aversion. If their aversion is severe enough to mean that mothers have to repeatedly de-latch their nurslings, or prematurely wean them off the breast entirely, they can feel that they have done something 'wrong' and, in doing so, harmed their nursling. Because a mother's love and the devotions of motherhood are epitomised as the most natural thing – the best way to be a mother – it is almost as if motherhood is reserved only for those who have done it 'correctly'. In history, single, unmarried mothers in the 18th century forfeited their right to this idealised motherhood by virtue of being poor and unwed and were openly ostracised and penalised. In literature there were distinct writings about *unnatural* mothers, or those who did not have the apparently natural instinct to mother. These were absent mothers, not-very-good mothers, or 'dead mothers' like those found in Jane Austen's works. Romanticised ideals of mothering persisted throughout the 19th century, but the reality was that – just like today – mothers were simply doing the best they could with what they had.

Breastfeeding took on the same narrative, because of the fundamental part it played in being a mother, and this is integral to our investigations into aversion. As milk-sharing dwindled, and the profession of wet nursing declined worldwide, modern families became nuclear and responsibility for breastfeeding landed squarely on a mother's shoulders. With new scientific research into breastfeeding linking it to brain development, and social theory moving away from behaviourism and linking the caregiver to the importance of attachment,* we begin to understand the concept of 'nurture'.

Breastfeeding as nursing: nursing as nurture

The word 'breastfeeding' literally describes the transference of milk through the breast when a nursling feeds. Mothers who struggle with aversion often mention the importance of breastmilk and breastfeeding, and many carry on

---

* Van der Horst, F. C. P., & van der Veer, R. (2008). Loneliness in Infancy: Harry Harlow, John Bowlby and Issues of Separation. *Integrative Psychological and Behavioural Science*, 42(4), 325–335.

breastfeeding despite the negative emotions they experience. But breastfeeding is more than just the transfer of milk. The word 'nursing' is often used synonymously with breastfeeding because it captures the aspect of care and nurture that the activity of breastfeeding entails. The word 'nurse' comes from the root meaning 'nourish', and by extension 'to care for', and more accurately describes what breastfeeding is: a holistic activity of mothering. What is of interest to us, but is not often talked about, is the impact aversion has on a mother's ability to *nurture*, essentially without the breast. If you are not a mother who is struggling with aversion right now, I have to tell you that this is harder than you might think, especially if breastfeeding was your go-to 'fix it' tool for pain, boredom, or comfort as your nursling got older. To further illustrate this point, I have turned to the Arabic language, which proves fascinating in terms of the interconnected parts of the root word for 'milk'. In Arabic all words have 'root' letters – three at most – from which linked 'stem' words are derived. The word 'milk' in Arabic is *halleeb* (حليب) and comes from the verb *halaba*, meaning to extract milk, and these words contain within them the root letters h (ح), l (ل), b (ب). Arabic dictionaries such as Hans Wehr and Lane's Lexicon list the many stems that come from the original root, amongst which are:

- To run, drip, trickle, ooze, leak (verb. *halaba*)
- To milk / milking (*halb*)
- Lactiferous (*halub*)
- To dream (*halama*)
- Dream (*hulm*)
- To be gentle, mild-tempered (*halīm*, pl. *haluma*)
- Patience, intelligence, reasoning (*hilm*, pl. *hulūm*/ *ahlām*)
- Nipple, teat, mammilla (*halam*)

Looking at these root words it is clear why the stem has links to both lactiferous and nipple. But *halaba* has a cluster of verbal meanings which are all directly interlinked and associated with not only milk, but also the consequences that the act of breastfeeding develops. Verbal stem links of *halaba* to patience, reasoning and to dream are interesting, and to intelligence as there is research linking breastfeeding to a higher IQ in children, showing more white brain matter. New research has also improved our understanding of the importance of neural development and secure attachment in the formative years.[*][**] We can see how bonds through breastfeeding affect not only health, but also a child's character and the ability to self-regulate emotions if they have had secure loving attachment growing up. In the Arabic language, a person who is intelligent is considered to be someone who can use their intellect to stabilise themselves in times of difficulty or tribulation: someone who can essentially self-regulate. Someone who does not lose their cool when things become stressful. An intelligent person, in this context, would not be disquieted by troubles. There are also many narratives in the predominant religion, Islam, linking milk and knowledge. To 'go astray', or not use your knowledge and ignore it in life (*ghawiya*), literally means an 'inability to digest milk'. In Islamic traditions, which are called *hadith*, milk and knowledge are often described as coming from the same source, and this was often interpreted to mean the qualities of milk itself somehow led to knowledge. A more relevant and accurate understanding based on recent research can lead to a different interpretation when considering 'breastfeeding' in a more holistic way, in the conceptual model of 'nurture'. It is very clear that in the Arabic language the word milk, and the act of breastfeeding has always been associated with more than just nourishment. This understanding would not be exclusive to the Arabs. Any nomadic or tribal peoples would have had a deep understanding of breastfeeding, what it brought to the community and how it benefited humans; it would have been symptomatic of what many pre-modern people understood. I think it would be a fascinating to do

---

[*]   Duhn, L. (2010). The Importance of Touch in the Development of Attachment. *Advances in Neonatal Care*, 10(6), 294.

[**]   Newman, L., Sivaratnam, C., & Komiti, A. (2015). Attachment and early brain development – neuroprotective interventions in infant–caregiver therapy. *Translational Developmental Psychiatry*, 3(1), 28647.

cross-cultural anthropological studies on the words used by non-industrialised, non-white communities to describe breastfeeding and milk. Research is already finding that, post-industrialisation, we are re-discovering what we as humans always knew – that breastmilk and breastfeeding is more than just food. It is not just the milk, but also the touch, the skinship that forms when breastfeeding that grows a nursling's body and brain (neuro-connection). It is not just the milk, but the responsiveness, the ability to respond to and quieten a nursling's cries through offering the breast, that develops a nursling's body and brain (responsive-reassurance).

There are also clear links in the root to stem connections between milk, intellect and dreaming: as mentioned before, the word to dream in Arabic is *halama*. The idea here is that it is hard to sleep peacefully (and consequently hard to dream) when you are agitated, stressed or perturbed. When a nursling is in a perturbed state, crying or in pain, mothers will put the infant to the breast, and one can visibly observe that the infant will go into a state of complete quietude and relaxation. Humans need this peace, this external quietude and internal reassurance, in order to sleep and therefore, to dream. Small humans are no different. A nursling with easy access to the nipple (*halam*) is literally instantly quieted because something is in its mouth, but also because hormones from the milk have sedative properties and bring relaxation, even reducing pain.[*] Herein lies the key understanding of breastfeeding as the main tool in our toolbox as mothers: we use it to calm, quiet, relax and soothe our babies, toddlers and children. And, crucially, to get nurslings to sleep. Bump? Breastfeed them. Tantrum? Breastfeed them. Teething? Breastfeed them. In pain? Breastfeed them. Overtired? Breastfeed them. Unwell? Breastfeed them. Getting vaccinated? Breastfeed them. The list is endless. Breastfeeding not only nourishes and grows our nurslings, it is also a formidable part of mothering as a whole, and thus being *able* to mother for breastfeeding

---

[*] Harrison, D., Reszel, J., Bueno, M., Sampson, M., Shah, V. S., Taddio, A., … Turner, L. (2016b). Breastfeeding for procedural pain in infants beyond the neonatal period. *The Cochrane Database of Systematic Reviews*, 10, CD011248.

women. When considering this, and the analysis of the Arabic words, it is difficult not to see the *activity* of breastfeeding in a much wider context of mothering – as direct caregiver responsiveness, as pain relief, as comfort, as part of the process of human nurture. When we talk of breastfeeding, we talk of an activity that is part of what it means to nurture as a mother. Figure 2 below illustrates this as a continuous positive cycle that allows mothers to nurture through to breastfeeding when aversion isn't present.

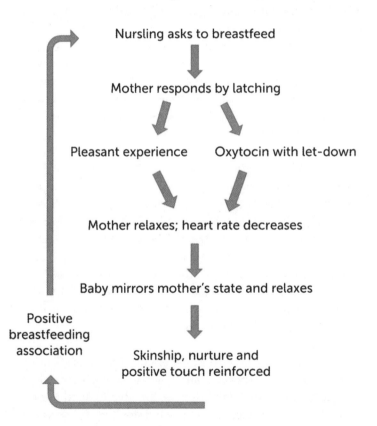

Breastfeeding Without Aversion

Nursling asks to breastfeed

Mother responds by latching

Pleasant experience   Oxytocin with let-down

Mother relaxes; heart rate decreases

Baby mirrors mother's state and relaxes

Positive breastfeeding association

Skinship, nurture and positive touch reinforced

Figure 2: Positive Association with Breastfeeding: Breastfeeding Without Aversion

Breastfeeding and negative associations

So what happens when aversion strikes? If it is severe, negative feelings may overwhelm the mother like an emotional hurricane, a force formidable enough to urge her to de-latch. Momentarily – and on one level unwillingly – she throws out the main tool in her toolbox. Imagine this has happened at 3am when she just cannot take one more second breastfeeding. De-latching may result in a crying nursling, who is unable to get back to sleep. This can (and does) create a bigger problem in the home. Imagine she has a sleeping toddler next to her, and cannot let her baby cry as it will wake them. Imagine this cycle continues for weeks, even months, daily. What happens to this breastfeeding relationship? What happens to nurture? What happens to a nursling who is unable to suckle as they are removed from the breast? What happens to a mother who is racked with guilt and shame because she cannot bear to breastfeed? The equilibrium at home is no longer there, and the bond established through skinship and breastfeeding begins to fragment.

> *Every feed I thought 'it would be different this time', and when she would ask for the breast I felt like I had purpose again . . . and on one level I wanted to feed her of course, she's my baby! Then, when she was on, it just felt so icky. I mean I could feel every drop being pulled out and the tongue ever so slightly on my nipple again and again. I just had rage. And when I couldn't bear it any longer, I would try to take her off. Of course then she would cry, and I would cry. And this just happened again and again. It was awful. It was such an awful time.* Hayling, Hong Kong

As mothers we know from experience that breastfeeding offers a unique, specific and literal connection when responding to a nursling's cries: we are able to soothe their discomfort, remove pain and in general stop the crying. There is a sense of relief, empowerment and purpose, all the while in skin-to-skin contact, sharing intimate warmth and movement with another little being.

Thanks to research in brain development and attachment theory we are now beginning to understand how and why this relationship is so important. For breastfeeding mothers and nurslings, their bond and secure attachment is built on this pattern of the mother offering breastfeeding to soothe the cries or pain of the nursling, from birth onwards. It may be all the nursling has known: the breast is a literal lifeline and a source of nourishment, contentment and love. Going back to the stories of neglect we mentioned earlier, there are theories that the 'first stage' of human development is to survive the first two years of life, or the 'first crisis' – and this requires not only feeding, but also the regulation of the infant's stress during this time. Mothers with aversion are often unable to offer this soothing to the degree they want to, or sometimes, to any degree at all. If aversion is persistent, it causes a problem that spreads out into the home environment and affects family dynamics and sleep. An unsettled nursling will often ask to breastfeed more, and a mother who practises nurturing through breastfeeding will respond by allowing suckling, but instead of breastfeeding resolving and improving the situation, breastfeeding with aversion actually makes it worse, as can be seen in Figure 3 on the next page, when mothers have a negative breastfeeding association because of their experience.[*]

The cure and the cause: the interwoven circles of bonding

The two concepts of skinship and nurture give us the foundations for what, I believe, makes aversion such an interesting – but heart-breaking – phenomenon for those who experience it. The dilemma for breastfeeding mothers who want to mother through breastfeeding is that the very same tool they have to mother, to create a bond, to quiet and console their infant, to have intimacy and skinship, is – with aversion – the very thing that is sabotaging those goals and the mother-nursling relationship. In these mothers, breastfeeding is both

---

[*] With thanks to insight from Anna Brauch, BA, IBCLC, LLLL.

Breastfeeding With Aversion:
The Vicious Cycle

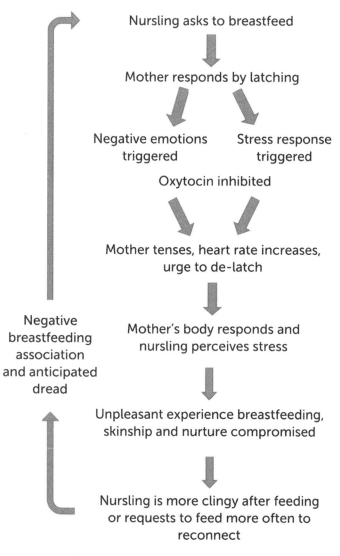

Nursling asks to breastfeed

Mother responds by latching

Negative emotions triggered

Stress response triggered

Oxytocin inhibited

Mother tenses, heart rate increases, urge to de-latch

Negative breastfeeding association and anticipated dread

Mother's body responds and nursling perceives stress

Unpleasant experience breastfeeding, skinship and nurture compromised

Nursling is more clingy after feeding or requests to feed more often to reconnect

Figure 3: Negative Association to Breastfeeding: Breastfeeding With Aversion

the cure and the cause of the situation. We know from decades of research the benefits of breastfeeding: that it protects both the mother and child against many diseases and conditions, but with aversion, instead of a win-win scenario for the mother and nursling, it turns into a zero-sum situation of sorts.[*] The nursling gains while the mother struggles and is impacted negatively when breastfeeding. The benefits become one-sided and the net benefit is zero, at least in the sense that the mother feels she is not benefiting from breastfeeding. In fact, she feels she is losing a great deal (time, bodily autonomy and so on, which we will cover later). Where does she get the notion that she is loosing a great deal? I believe, in the expectation of what normal breastfeeding is supposed to be like.

The myth of 'normal' breastfeeding emotions

There is an assumption in this book that mothers with aversion are 'struggling', and wrestle with controlling negative emotions. Implicit in this struggle is the notion that many women consider what they are feeling to be 'wrong', and they do not identify with the person they have become when they experience aversion. In my study, women even stated that they are confused about why they get aversion: it is often both unexpected and unwelcome. Before delving into what aversion is in detail in the next chapter, I want to address 'normal' breastfeeding: what it looks like, how it ought to feel, and what emotions are attributed to it. Most research efforts into breastfeeding have looked at the first few months of a baby's life to six months – and look at the importance and impact of *exclusive* breastfeeding. Despite an explosion of research into infant feeding and human breastmilk, there is still so much to be learnt about the newborn period that research into breastfeeding older nurslings has very much fallen by the wayside. Consequently, mothers' and nurslings' challenges

---

[*]   Simply when a gain for one side entails a corresponding loss for the other. Collins English Dictionary. (n.d.). Retrieved 5 September 2019, from www.collinsdictionary.com/dictionary/english/zero-sum-game

and emotions when breastfeeding past the newborn stage are rarely studied. So, for now, we need a little common sense to get us though.

What is a 'normal' breastfeeding experience?

Breastfeeding can be joyful: at the beginning, throughout a breastfeeding journey, at different stages, or not at all for some women. It can be a burden, during the intensive newborn feeding stage, or throughout, intermittently at stages, or never really a burden for some women. Some women love breastfeeding at the beginning, at different periods, or even most of the time; others actually positively hate it. Others still are indifferent; it is just something they 'do'. Breastfeeding can be painful: not just at the beginning, but intermittently at different stages of the breastfeeding journey or even continuously for some women. The condition of Raynaud's when breastfeeding is a good example of that, or, as in my own case, sensitive nipples and breastfeeding nurslings with restrictive tongue-ties, which meant constant palate contact for me and my poor nipples. Ouch. Some mothers start their journey with formula feeding or using a supplemental nursing system. Others may be cup-feeding, use nipple shields or express and bottle feed – the latter especially at a midway point because of a life event or the need to return to work. Other mothers will use one or more of these methods for their entire feeding journey. While some of us take pride in our infant feeding path, others find the infant feeding method shameful and feel a failure. With all of these observations, can you see what I am getting at? There is no 'normal' breastfeeding experience, nor normal breastfeeding-related emotions, or feelings attributed to it that are 'right'. There is a spectrum of experiences, and a wide range of emotions. My own breastfeeding experience made me consider not what a good breastfeeding journey was, but what substantiates a good breastfeeding *relationship*. Was it the exclusivity of breastfeeding, was it the duration, was it that you enjoyed it, was it that you responded and offered the breast when your child needed it? Was it that you never experienced negative thoughts or emotions when breastfeeding? It could be all of these, or none of them. What constitutes a good relationship is not set, except by the mother's own expectations of what breastfeeding will be like, her personal goals and her experience of it. For some women, becoming a breastfeeding mother is very much culturally determined, while for others it is a personally set and determined goal. For the experience, I believe it is precisely in the *expectation* of what breastfeeding *should* be like that the misunderstanding lies. What breastfeeding is in reality is often not as we expect. And consequently, the experience of aversion will seem misplaced in a breastfeeding journey if a mother gets it. Somehow wrong. Somehow an aberration.

This mistake is also a mistake of language and how it is used. We understand the word 'normal' to mean what usually happens most of the time, which may be the case in reality, and so an accurate way to describe something. But we then turn this usual occurrence into what should happen all of the time: it becomes turned into what is 'proper' and thus desirable. It becomes about the correct way to be, and the correct way to feel. And even though the emotions we will be focusing on in this book are generally understood as 'negative' emotions, it is a myth to think of emotions related to breastfeeding as belonging in only two groups – 'positive' and 'negative' – and that one is 'normal' and the other 'abnormal'. One 'good', and the other 'bad'. Rather, it could be said that to one degree or another both these types of emotions, in varying proportions, are present in everybody, at different times. The 'negative' ones may indicate something is wrong, or that something needs to change, but that is not to say that if you do experience them that it is somehow abnormal. On the contrary, one study shows that feeling angry is good for you and can even make you happier. According to Dr Maya Tamir, who was the lead researcher of the study, anger and hatred can actually make you happy because when we feel useful emotions, even if they may be unpleasant to experience, we can start to regulate them in strategic ways to our benefit.[*] The point is, if you allow

---

[*] Ford, B.Q., & Tamir, M. (2012). When getting angry is smart: Emotional preferences and emotional intelligence. *Emotion*, *12*(4), 685–689.

yourself to feel emotions that are arising, and you want to feel them, regardless of whether they are pleasant or unpleasant, then you are more emotionally intelligent, and consequently you are better off. Basically, if you are okay with getting angry then you will feel better and happier than someone who feels awful about it.

The problem, however, is that when the phenomenon of aversion is being experienced, there is compromised *parent-infant reciprocity* during feeding, whether it be the mother resenting having to feed at that time and getting angry inside, or whether there are visible negative emotions and physical de-latching of the nursling. The reciprocity withers away and it becomes a one-way relationship in many senses: the nursling suckles, the nursling 'gains'. Whether it is due to the frequency of requests, frequency of feeds, behaviour and temperament when refused feeds or the number of night-time wakings to feed, many mothers feel stuck between a rock and a hard place when aversion strikes. We fear the harm we may do if we refuse our nurslings – or wean before our nurslings are ready – and we feel immense guilt at the thought of not being a responsive 'good' mother. As we are born into an age of scientific research, with the cult of maternity, we cannot shake our identity as mothers from the idealised mothers we believe to be normal, obtainable. When experiencing aversion, mothers feel as if they have failed as mothers because they are *breastfeeding mothers*, and are attached to their nurslings. The negative emotions are an internal pressure, a force that is there to drive you to take action. Depending on the severity of aversion and the length of time it is experienced, it is only a matter of time before the mother is worn down from the attrition of experiencing it, and her negative emotions 'leak' – whether this is by crying, shouting or de-latching. This spill-over can cause the vicious cycle of aversion to kick in because emotional states are contagious. Emotional mirroring, and emotional projection, are common in other situations: negative emotions can be 'caught.'* This means that a mother's reaction to aversion and the way she deals

---

* Parkinson, B. (2011). Interpersonal Emotion Transfer: Contagion and Social Appraisal. *Interpersonal Emotion Transfer*, 5, 428–439.

with stress will affect the nursling, and in turn the nursling's response to the mother's negative emotions will be affected. How we outwardly react when we experience aversion may seem reasonable, and when rationalising the situation, as we will see later on in the book, but reacting can make the situation worse. This is true of many situations outside of aversion. I have seen mothers who are fearful of the pain from damaged nipples, tensing their shoulders up when trying to latch their nursling, thus compromising the positioning of the latch and therefore the attachment of the nursling, making the latch worse. This, in turn, makes the pain worse. Yet, at the time of difficulty, how are they to know they are making it worse? And how could we as mothers *stop* reacting in a time of difficulty or pain? It can be very difficult to make objective decisions and assess a situation you are in without external support, which is often the case for breastfeeding mothers.[*] It is very difficult not to react, or not to try to take steps to resolve or rectify a situation. I have seen mothers who are clinically hyper-lactating, but who only see that their baby is fussy and unsettled after a 20-minute feed and think they are hungry again because they do not have enough milk. So, to resolve this situation, the mothers start pumping to make more milk, and in doing so make everything much worse. What do we do when a challenge or problem hits us, whether perceived or real? We tend to take *action*, but without realising it could compound our problems. We will *try* to make it better, as it is our instinct to try, because as humans we tend to move away from stress, discomfort or pain. And as breastfeeding mothers we do so for good reason. Amir and colleagues actually demonstrated a correlation between breastfeeding pain and maternal stress, and showed that depression scores normalised as breastfeeding difficulties were resolved.[**]

Remember, breastfeeding and breastmilk are good. Stress,

---

*   Fox, R., McMullen, S., & Newburn, M. (2015). UK women's experiences of breastfeeding and additional breastfeeding support: A qualitative study of Baby Café services. *BMC Pregnancy and Childbirth, 15*.

**   Buck, M.L., Amir, L.H., Cullinane, M., & Donath, S.M. (2013). Nipple Pain, Damage, and Vasospasm in the First 8 Weeks Postpartum. *Breastfeeding Medicine, 9*(2), 56–62.

not so good. I have often wondered about Katie Hinde's work, in which she shows that cortisol in milk and infant temperament is linked in primates. If the mother is stressed, the nursling picks up stress hormones. Is it the case that negative emotions in mothers with aversion will affect a nursling whether they 'spill over' or not? Does experiencing aversion, or being stressed when breastfeeding, especially persistently, mean your nursling's behaviour changes? Hinde found in a study of rhesus macaques that the milk of the mother could affect the behaviour of the infant because it contributed to the development of the brain, and so the behavioural dispositions the infant had. Although the study was in another mammal, the data indicates that there may be mechanisms for what the authors call 'nutritional programming' – a fancy way to describe how the milk transferred affects infant temperament and the development of behaviour in response to maternal or environmental conditions.* It is not much of a stretch to say that the mother's behaviour and emotions, as well as the milk itself, are implicated in the infant's response when aversion strikes.**

---

*   Ibid.

**   Hinde, K., & Capitanio, J.P. (2010). Lactational programming? Mother's milk energy predicts infant behavior and temperament in rhesus macaques (Macaca mulatta). *American Journal of Primatology, 72*(6), 522–529.

PART II

The Cure and
The Cause

3

Aversion: The Phenomenon

What do we know about aversion?

One of the first books I read that mentioned experiencing negative emotions when breastfeeding was by Hilary Flower. In 2000, in the first edition of *Adventures in Tandem Nursing*, Flower writes that some women can experience 'agitation' when breastfeeding through pregnancy, but as I read the book, it didn't help me understand why I had experienced aversion when I only had one child. From then on I was only able to find blogs with personal stories about aversion and so I prepared my own survey to research it a bit more. While I was sifting through hundreds and hundreds of responses to my questionnaire about aversion in 2016, Watkinson and her colleagues published a paper in which they had interviewed women about their breastfeeding experiences, concluding that 'breastfeeding has the potential to trigger a range of conflicting cognitions and emotions in mothers that may impact on how mothers view themselves and relate to their children'.* This was a groundbreaking article for me, and it spurred me to continue my research on aversion for this book.

In 2017 I published a paper on a qualitative study I conducted that described the phenomenon of aversion using mothers' own words and terms, in which I identified themes of onset, duration and severity that arose from the data I

---

* Watkinson, M., Murray, C., & Simpson, J. (2016). Maternal experiences of embodied emotional sensations during breast feeding: An Interpretative Phenomenological Analysis. *Midwifery, 36*, 53–60.

collected.* Along with a whole lot of work to raise awareness on social media, it was clear by now that negative emotions can, and are, triggered by breastfeeding for many women. I began to think about the causes of aversion a lot more after this because there were so many unanswered questions, and so many women who struggled. I started to think that even if breastfeeding is triggering these emotions, this doesn't mean breastfeeding alone is necessarily causing them. I thought about traditional mothering in modern-day society, and the conflicts and challenges that could present. I wondered about my own experience of aversion, and how physical pain or physical conditions can affect breastfeeding. In 2018, I presented at the Breastfeeding and Feminism Conference in North Carolina on how maternal autonomy and consent may be compromised when experiencing aversion, exploring difficulties with body boundaries and the feeling of being 'touched out'. The abstract of this was published later that year in the *Journal of Human Lactation*.** Later that year a paper suggested that naturopathic support, including taking nutritional supplements or herbal remedies, may help with aversion in mothers who are tandem feeding.*** And a case report by McGuire suggests that even though mothers are motivated to breastfeed, aversion could be an indicator to wean.**** Since then there have been a few more articles published, and I have no doubt that there will be many more in years to come as interest in this area of research increases.

* Yate, Z. (2017). A qualitative study on negative emotions triggered by breastfeeding; Describing the phenomenon of breastfeeding/nursing aversion and agitation in breastfeeding mothers. *Iranian Journal of Nursing and Midwifery Research*, 22(6), 449.

** 13th Breastfeeding and Feminism International Conference: The Dance of Nurture in a Complex World: How Biology, Gender, and Social Context Shape How We Nourish Our Children. Maternal autonomy and challenges of consent in mothers who experience the phenomenon of breastfeeding/nursing aversion and agitation: an internal ethical conflic (2018). *Journal of Human Lactation*, 34(3), 600–630.

*** Steel, A. (2018). Naturopathic support for nursing aversion associated with tandem breastfeeding. *Australian Journal of Herbal and Naturopathic Medicine*, 30(2), 74

**** McGuire, E. (2018). Breastfeeding aversion and agitation. *Breastfeeding Review*, 26(2), 37

The nitty-gritty horribleness

Aversion is when women can experience particular negative emotions like anger, agitation and irritation, and certain intrusive thoughts like feeling like a 'prisoner', feeling 'violated' or thoughts of pushing or throwing the child 'across the room' when their nursling is *latched*. If you know exactly what I mean, then I'm sure you feel the relief washing over you as you read that. It's a thing. If you don't know what I mean, and you don't understand what kind of mother would think something like that, I urge you not to be alarmed – leave that to the women who experience these thoughts, seemingly out of nowhere, and are overwhelmed with guilt and shame afterwards. The activity of breastfeeding clearly triggers some very unpleasant emotions and breastfeeding itself can become the cause of anxiety and stress in some breastfeeding mothers:

> *Y'know, sometimes I just didn't want to breastfeed, I just wanted to hug him okay if he hurt himself or if he woke up at night. But no, it was like there was never a time he could be near me without reaching inside my top for titty. It got to me y'know? I just started stressin' every time he got close.*
> Felisha, Colorado

As some mothers report experiencing aversion when pumping, I am inclined to believe it is not just suckling at the breast by a nursling, but also the activity of milk extraction and physical contact with the breast that is in question when we try to understand aversion:

> *I was at work one day pumping and I got this wave of anger. I wanted to stop pumping, I wanted to stop it right now. I was feeling fine before I got there but then I was super-annoyed, out of nowhere. It really put a downer on my day.* Beatrice, Texas

Mothers can have a paroxysm of negative emotions when experiencing aversion. Don't worry, I had to look that word up too when I first read it. Paroxysm as a noun can be used to describe a sudden uncontrollable outburst, ie, paroxysms of rage. I thought it quite appropriate to use, even though I am still not 100% sure how to pronounce it, as it's a very accurate description of how aversion 'spills over' and a mother cannot suppress her negative feelings. This emotional outburst, particularly if it happens frequently, is one of the main causes of guilt that follows, especially after de-latching. In its essence, this paroxysm of anger is the character antithesis of the loving mother we consider or identify ourselves to be (given what we are told mothers *should* be like). If you are not able to control yourself, or you behave in a way you deem inappropriate, then you can feel as though you are letting your nursling down by not being the type of mother they need. Mothers feel that they are letting themselves down too, by caving in and reacting to negative emotions or acting on them. This struggle of the 'will' to do something, and the 'weakness' of that will to follow it through is a theme we find in the phenomenon of aversion. The will is something that allows a mother to continue breastfeeding through aversion, considering it often means she has an urge to stop breastfeeding. Particularly in a mother who struggles with persistent aversion and who wants to continue to breastfeed, or, even if she has decided she really does not want to continue, her nursling clearly does want to. Ideally, weaning is a *process* and there are two parties involved in that process in order to make it a smooth one. Regardless, it is not always easy, nor the right option, to 'just wean' from breastfeeding, despite what people will say:

Why can't I just wean? Well, she cries and screams and that makes me feel sad. And what about when she is poorly and she can't eat? What would I do? It is not as simple as that [weaning]. Panteh, New Orleans

This kind of story was frequent in my data from the mothers' responses in my study. It took me a long time to read through all the mothers' stories from my research as they were so heartfelt, and so many said they hadn't before told anyone how they felt or what was happening. When I was reading them I found some recognisable patterns of when aversion started in women, how long it carried on for, and how severe it was. The most surprising aspect to me was that the feelings and thoughts described were very similar, from mothers of different demographic statuses and in different parts of the world. I had mothers from Africa, Australia, Bahrain, Canada, France, Germany, India, Iran, the UK and the US. For many mothers there was a feeling of physical repulsion when breastfeeding, while for others it was to do with a lack of body autonomy. Some mothers mentioned that they experienced it more severely when their mind was on something else and they were not concentrating on breastfeeding their nursling because they wanted to be somewhere else or doing something else. Many hadn't told anyone because they thought something was wrong with them:

> *I am not very sure how to say it, but feeding her is making me angry right now. I know it shouldn't, maybe this is not normal, and I need some kind of help, but it is how I feel. I want to take her off my breast.* Priya, Lahore

Some mothers attributed aversion to their life becoming stressful, or feeling very rundown, while others only experienced it when they were sleep deprived. Despite their own theories on why they experienced aversion, the emotional load was often written about too, with guilt attached to the feelings and shame in how they manifested. And despite a variety of stories and attributed causes, there were several very common self-reported symptoms of aversion.

Symptoms of aversion

Symptoms are often used to classify a condition or disease in medicine, and they are subjective and self-reported. They are different from medical signs, which are objective and testable. Symptoms are a physical manifestation, an indication that something – often undesirable – exists. It's helpful to think of mothers' descriptions of aversion in terms of symptoms, because women often see a change in themselves, something different happening, when aversion strikes. Symptoms are often a reaction to some kind of change, whether biological, physical, mental or emotional. Symptoms can be grouped into categories, and you can experience some and not all of them. If you have a cluster of symptoms from the following list, it is likely that you too are experiencing aversion.

- Dreading a feed or anxiety about having to feed.
- Anger or rage when a nursling is latched.
- Agitation or irritability when a nursling is latched.
- Skin itching/skin-crawling sensation when a nursling is latched.
- Self-harming when breastfeeding in order to continue feeding.
- Overwhelming urge to de-latch a nursling.
- Feeling violated, or 'used'.
- Feeling like you have not consented to being touched when a nursling is latched.
- Feelings of guilt about the negative emotions.
- Feelings of shame about the negative emotions.
- Thoughts of wanting to self-harm.
- Thoughts of wanting to 'push the nursling off' or 'throw the infant across the room'.
- Thoughts of feeling trapped or like a prisoner because of having to breastfeed.
- Thoughts of hating breastfeeding.

When do these symptoms start showing? Well, aversion can strike at any point in a breastfeeding journey, from the very start at birth, or seemingly 'out of nowhere' a few years into the breastfeeding journey. I vividly remember the day a lady messaged me for support via the aversion resource site. She had six children, and had breastfed each one for many months, some even years, and had never experienced aversion. She was months into breastfeeding her sixth child when aversion hit. She was shocked, saddened and beside herself:

I've been breastfeeding for nearly 18 years; it's never not been a part of what I do every day. I'm a mom, and I have breastfed all my children. My youngest is nine months old, and all of a sudden I just feel like I have had enough. I can't bear to do another feed, I'm so irritated when my baby is latched onto me, and it has become hard to just sit and breastfeed. I have no clue what is happening to me.
Sheila, Brisbane

Some women can link aversion to their postnatal menses returning, or to their monthly menses; others know it happens specifically on the days when they ovulate. This kind of hormonal link to the experience is also found by those who experience it when breastfeeding through pregnancy. It is known that around two-thirds of women experience agitation when feeding through pregnancy, along with milk 'drying up', and changes in nipple sensitivity.

First time round, I got aversion when I fell pregnant, guess my milk dried up and the dry sucking really hurt my nipples. With my second though I started getting it when he was 15 months old and turned into a total boobie-monster. Freya, Norwich

Aside from aversion in pregnancy, which often disappears once the baby is born and the milk 'comes in', we do not yet know why aversion goes away for some mothers who struggle, but doesn't for others. Women may experience aversion only once; others experience it at every feed, even from when their baby is a newborn. There is a variation in how long it lasts, and it is not clear exactly why it starts in some dyads.

I got this antsy feeling when I was breastfeeding a few weeks ago, felt like creepy crawlies under my skin, I couldn't shake it until he had finished feeding. It hasn't happened since but I hope it doesn't happen again, it wasn't nice. Mona, California

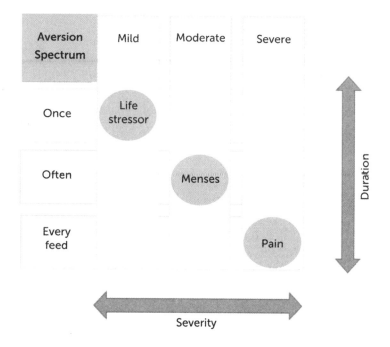

Figure 4: The Aversion Spectrum: Onset, Severity and Duration

Spectrum of aversion

Figure 4 shows how mothers can experience aversion at different times, and in differing severities. Mothers can also move between these areas as the breastfeeding journey progresses. Whether women experience mild aversion a couple of times when going through a life stressor, or whether they have severe aversion at every feed, the symptoms reported are similar.

A lot of mothers also describe a skin-crawling sensation, which is known as *formication* in medical literature. This is a peculiar type of sensation that is often described as feeling like small insects crawling under the skin, and its cause is often attributed to our nerves, depending on the condition. It is actually a well-known symptom of medical conditions like Parkinson's disease and multiple sclerosis. Although I am not saying that this symptom has any link to those conditions in nursing mothers, the feeling may have links to a nerve response in those women that experience it as part of aversion. If you are in an aversion support group online, you will see many posts that mention formication:

> *Does anyone else feel like they have insects crawling under their skin when breastfeeding? I want to itch my skin so badly it's doing my head it, I don't know what to do. He's 13 months.*
> Laura, Blackpool

> *I have had it [aversion] with singletons and twins. The worst was feeding my son when I was pregnant with my daughter. I used to lie there feeding him to sleep, giving him comfort whilst my skin crawled and I fantasised about somehow being able to split my skin open and slide out of it to escape.*
> Ophelia, Geneva

Other women talk about a neuralgia-type feeling when their infant is latched and aversion kicks in. Neuralgia is a nerve pain thought to be caused by nerve damage, irritation or inflammation. Such unpleasant or abnormal sensations when being touched are called dysesthesia. I have often wondered whether these sensations indicate the role of the nervous system in the experience of aversion for these women. Unfortunately, anecdotal data and reports from women who experience aversion are not enough to understand this part of aversion, but one day there will be research into why some women experience these particular feelings when their nursling is latched:

> *If I could tell someone what kind of tornado is whirling around in my body when I have to nurse her, they would think I was crazy. I swear my skin starts burning up with pain, I want to rip it off . . . I'm all of a sudden vehemently angry. All I want to do is get my baby off me, and now.* Jennifer, Oxford

Not all women experience such severe aversion, or feel a paroxysm of rage. Women also report experiencing aversion in a milder form, without anger or rage, but with irritation and agitation when their nursling latches. And while this may seem easier for the mother, they too have triggers for their aversion, an urge to de-latch, and the subsequent waves of both guilt and shame. Guilt says we have done something wrong, shame says there is something wrong with us; and they are closely aligned. If we are prone to shame, we can feel guilty easily even if it is not a 'true' guilt (hating breastfeeding and de-latching if you are in pain should not really make you feel guilty). Guilt can also mature into disgust, which we can see arise in aversion too. The negative emotions that characterise aversion can plague the breastfeeding activity, cause strong negative associations and take considerable effort to combat. Aversion, regardless of where mothers find themselves on the severity spectrum, will create an emotional burden on the mother, and invariably can affect the family home dynamic.

> *When I got aversion I found that breastfeeding was becoming so unbearable an activity for me that I couldn't hide it. My poor girl seeing her mum like that . . . I guess it made her feel anxious and she started acting out, especially when she would ask for num nums and I would be saying 'no' or 'not right now' all the time. It made being at home with her impossible.*
> Abigail, Berlin

Hey, isn't this Dysphoric Milk Ejection Reflex? (D-MER)

The short answer is no; I don't think it is. If you haven't heard of the condition D-MER, it is characterised by a wave of negative feelings like hopelessness, despair and homesickness for a few minutes while the milk lets down, and there is very little known about it.[*] Lots of women with D-MER also experience the negative feelings of aversion, like anger, agitation and

---

[*] Ureño, T.L., Buchheit, T. L., Hopkinson, S. G., & Berry-Cabán, C. S. (2018). Dysphoric Milk Ejection Reflex: A Case Series. *Breastfeeding Medicine: The Official Journal of the Academy of Breastfeeding Medicine*, 13(1), 85-88.

irritation, but I believe the two are distinct. One of the main differences is that if you have D-MER, which you will be able to self-identify, the feelings dissipate, or 'go away', during a feed. The feelings connected to D-MER generally subside within 10 minutes, because they are linked to the milk release, whereas with aversion they will last the *whole time the infant is latched*, whether that is 20 minutes or the two-hour bedtime feed. Another distinction is that the negative feelings are rather different. Anger and rage are not homesickness and despair, and anyone who experiences both D-MER and aversion will attest to this. However, I do think the two are interlinked, and if you experience D-MER, you are more prone to experience aversion due to the added distress, emotional difficulty and anxiety when breastfeeding that D-MER can create. Heise, who published the original paper on D-MER, hypothesised the role of prolactin and dopamine in the condition.[*] Recently, Kendall-Tackett and Moberg proposed an oxytocin-related mechanism, suggesting that as the feelings dissipate in under 10 minutes they are unlikely be caused by prolactin, as levels don't start rising until 10 minutes into a feed. They put forward a theory suggesting that oxytocin is abnormally upregulating a mother's stress response: triggering the fight or flight response instead of the calm, loving feeling it is known for. The normal way the mechanism pathway works is that when stress is up, oxytocin is down. Yet in D-MER, as oxytocin is released it seems to be upregulating a stress response.[**],[***] In recognising similarities and differences, I do think that part of the aversion experience for some mothers is rooted in the same hormone, oxytocin, and that an upregulated stress response occurs when aversion strikes, but this response doesn't explain the whole

[*] Heise, A.M. (2017). *Before the letdown: Dysphoric milk ejection reflex and the breastfeeding mother.* [Independently published].

[**] Uvnas-Moberg, K., & Kendall-Tackett, K. (2018). The Mystery of D-MER: What Can Hormonal Research Tell Us About Dysphoric Milk-Ejection Reflex? *Clinical Lactation, 9*(1), 23–29.

[***] Uvnäs-Moberg, K., Ekström-Bergström, A., Berg, M., Buckley, S., Pajalic, Z., Hadjigeorgiou, E., … Dencker, A. (2019). Maternal plasma levels of oxytocin during physiological childbirth – a systematic review with implications for uterine contractions and central actions of oxytocin. *BMC Pregnancy and Childbirth, 19*(1), 285.

experience of aversion. I would argue that a mother's biological responses vary because of other factors, often external, and that aversion is likely to happen particularly if the stress response is persistently triggered in some women when breastfeeding, because of a vicious cycle as shown in Figure 2 on page 33. A breastfeeding mother who is responsive, who is in charge of the wellbeing and sustenance of her nursling, will take this position seriously. If she doesn't respond to a nursling's cue for milk, or comfort, she will feel she is in violation of her covenant as a mother, who by the very definition of a mother as she understands it cannot withhold care. Yet being triggered and getting aversion can make responding to the needs of her nursling very challenging, particularly when the nursling's temperament is demanding or overwhelming, or in direct conflict with the mother's personal preferences and needs. Thus, aversion becomes the manifestation of not only biology, and societal pressure, but also a kind of learned behaviour: breastfeeding becomes a negatively associated experience. This can happen for a number of reasons, which we will cover in the next chapter.

4

Conflict and Preferences

'Touched out' and other triggers

Triggers are catalysts that cause a reaction and they usually happen just before aversion kicks in. The number of triggers women report are varied, but have particular themes and I have grouped them into the following areas: sensation and touch, sleep interruption and deprivation, and what I call 'conditional breastfeeding', which refers to breastfeeding that becomes overbearingly restrictive, but is often necessary for home peace and balance. This list of triggers is by no means comprehensive, and I expect more to be revealed as research into aversion continues. They are not standalone triggers as they overlap, and they are also specific to the mother, or mother and nursling pair – meaning what are triggers for some are not for others. The first set of triggers are related to the initial chapter and the importance of touch that builds relationships, and touch that doesn't. Being 'touched out' is a common phrase mothers use, and a main trigger for many women.

> *I personally felt 'touched out' – like I never had my own space – and it created nursing aversion for me. Don't get me wrong I loved feeding and I am so glad I did, if I had another I hope I could feed again, but I was ready to stop after three years.*
> Sarah, Kampala

Sensation and touch

Sexual arousal when breastfeeding is not abnormal – although many breastfeeding mothers may think it is, or feel embarrassed that they become aroused. In the field of lactivism we like to stress the fact that breasts aren't sex organs. We say that breasts are only there to feed our young – as breasts have mammary glands – to combat society's taboo on breastfeeding in public because of 'indecent exposure', or the ridiculous assertion that women 'do it to get attention'. However, it also remains a fact that breasts and nipples are sensitive areas, stimulate orgasms and are very much involved in sexual relations. The sensation of a nursling's suckling on the breast can be little different to a partner doing so, but for some women this causes sensory pleasure, even orgasm. When breastfeeding women have what they think are inappropriate feelings, they can feel embarrassed and ashamed and want to suppress them in order to continue feeding. When they cannot suppress them, aversion can manifest. It is a sort of angry frustration about not wanting to feel the way she does, and not wanting to feel that way when she is touched or being suckled on because of the need to separate sexual feelings from her nursling.

Breastfeeding is not a lot like sex, but intimacy in space and touch, with body-to-body contact, necessarily happens when breastfeeding and in sexual relations, in quite sensitive areas of the body. It's reasonable to think that, just like sex, individual people have individual preferences about what kinds of touch and sensation they like and do not like. For example, most women are not irked by the idea of a towel brushing over their nipples when coming out of the shower, but for a small proportion of women even the *idea* of this makes them shudder – particularly post-lactogenesis when nipples are constantly erect. Touch is so important in relationships, but so is the right kind of touch. You may think that stroking is always a nice touch; it's soft and relaxing, what's not to like? Yet, for some women who are breastfeeding, stroking is the absolute last thing they want when they have been climbed on, sucked on, touched, and tugged at all day, and possibly all night too. Stroking becomes just another sensation of touch that they don't want. Breastfeeding is contact enough, and it takes great strength at times to tolerate – with all the movement, the noise and sensation of suckling, the irritation of nipples when flutter suckling happens, and the hot sweaty ear or the weight of a partially-sleeping nursling. All of these things – or some in combination – require formidable patience to be able to endure for an ongoing period of time for some.

So now we have some context, it is very clear from stories of mothers with aversion that breastfeeding women are contending with some or all of the following antics:

1. Nipple tweaking/twiddling (twisting, pulling, hitting, flicking, or stroking the nipple that isn't latched on to).
2. Scratching.
3. Pinching.
4. Stroking.
5. Wandering hands.
6. Punching.
7. Excessive infant body movement (to paint this picture more clearly, this often results in movement *away* from the breast while still *attached to* the breast).

We all have different thresholds of comfortable touch so it is unsurprising that for some these are triggers for aversion. Other factors, such as how healthy or poorly mothers are, how much internal or external stress they feel, or simply with how tired they feel, may also contribute.

Sleep disturbance and sleep deprivation

I was always a night owl as a child, which made getting up for school quite hard, and this didn't change as I grew up. I never made the 9am lectures at university, and I would always seem to work better at night. The 9–5 working days post-university were a struggle for me and I never enjoyed the early morning wakes, even a decade later when I became a mother. I had my first baby, and as you do when you don't know better, I listened to all the advice about getting babies *into a routine* and put my nursling *to bed early*. This was mainly to get a grip on my first-born's seemingly erratic (but now understood as biologically normal) waking. And we are still entrenched in this routine six years later, as he consistently wakes between 5.30 and 6am – though thankfully the number of night wakings has drastically reduced. Looking back, I am not sure any of our interventions to get him to sleep better actually ended up making any difference to his sleep. As he got older, he just slept a little deeper, a little longer, a little better. The only sure thing the interventions did was ensure he woke early, meaning I had to keep getting up between 4 and 5am – which kind of killed me. Especially, when he would wake every 45 minutes to an hour every night to breastfeed as well. And I was not alone in struggling with all this sleep-related palaver and its consequences.

Sleep is such a complex factor in motherhood that I do wonder if aversion would even exist if breastfeeding mothers got the sleep they need. But sleep interruptions are necessarily part of the night-time responsive care that all nurslings need, the relationship between sleep and negative feelings when breastfeeding has not been properly studied. So for now we must rely on mothers' own reports about how sleep interruptions add to their aversion, make it worse, or are the actual trigger for their aversion. Some of the things they mention include:

1. Cluster feeding in the early part of the night (typically in the newborn period, but also at times of teething, sickness and developmental growth spurts).
2. Nurslings who are literally latched on all night (sleeping with a breast in their mouth).
3. Nurslings who need to breastfeed/re-latch to fall back asleep (day naps or night sleep).
4. Frequent wakes to breastfeed at night.
5. Constant contact, touch and movement at night, particularly if bed-sharing.

Any of these can affect the number of hours and the quality of sleep a mother gets. This is not to mention the mental attrition that can occur when responding to the needs of a nursling to suckle. This book does not debate whether a nursling actually 'needs' to suckle or not, but rather aims to catalogue the instances when they do and a mother finds it tiresome, to the extent that it can trigger aversion. Waking to feed a newborn every two hours may seem tiresome, but many mothers can tolerate it, knowing it is a necessity to ensure the growth of their nursling. Waking every two hours to feed a two-year-old is another story entirely, and requires a greater mental effort to endure. This leads us into the psychological aspect that affects the triggers for aversion.

Conditional breastfeeds

Breastfeeding is not often a kinetic activity for the mother. What I mean to say is that although one *can* do it while moving, such as in a rocking chair, or with a baby in a sling, breastfeeding as an activity is not about movement. There is actually a lot of non-movement for the mother with breastfeeding, especially when trying to get nurslings to sleep for naps or at bedtime. Non-movement accumulates, with time spent feeding multiple times during the night, or whenever nurslings are unwell or teething. When contact napping, or at night-time, mothers feel the weight of this non-movement because there are no distractions. There are no other people around and they can start to feel the pressure of being trapped in the room because there is no other way to get their nursling to sleep. Often, there is no other person who can step in to help them:

> He never took a bottle, to a snuggy, or to my husband for that matter. He will only fall asleep without boob when there is some kind of movement in a car or pushchair – so it's just me getting him to sleep and back to sleep at night. It's lonely, yes, but what's more is it's unbearably suffocating because I feel trapped in that room. Charlotte, Kampala

You could argue that the reality of 'being trapped in a room at night' is not as dire as breastfeeding mothers make out. It's just half an hour or an hour of the night when they have to wait until their nursling sleeps and they can have time for themselves. Perhaps this may be factually true, but it is missing the point. Whether you perceive or actually experience the activity of breastfeeding as restrictive doesn't matter, because of the burden felt from being the nursling's sole caregiver, and the fact that the nursling is totally reliant and dependent on you. Mothers who breastfeed this way are *always* on call, for every re-settle, every illness, every sleep time, every fall, every request. Every minute. This is enough to affect many women, especially those who take an attachment parenting approach to mothering, who realise the importance of nurture and have seen the benefits of skinship. These mothers may feel a sense of duty, or obligation, and that their nursling's growth and success in life is dependent on them 'getting it right', and that part of this is to breastfeed. This kind of mothering takes time to get used to, and frankly, some mothers never quite get used to this level of responsibility, perhaps because so few have known anything about it before becoming a mother.* Or perhaps many mothers are not prepared for it because, as a topic, it is eerily lacking in our mandatory education systems, or because many of us live in societies that reinforce false myths about babies and motherhood in order to sell you products. Whichever it is, the experience of feeling physically constrained when breastfeeding, and mentally accepting that you are solely depended on, is an important factor in the psychological portion of aversion.

I want to make it clear at this point that it is biologically normal for an infant to be 'dependent' on their mother and breastfeeding to fall asleep, and there is nothing actually *wrong* with a baby or toddler being dependant on the breast to sleep. Nor is there anything wrong when a mother is herself dependant on using the breast to get her nursling to sleep – we all know it can be the fastest and easiest way – and that's probably because nature designed it that way. Human milk has sedative properties, and the mother is a source of comfort and security: a combination that means suckling at the breast

---

*   We cover this point later in Chapter 6.

is often the best place for a vulnerable small human being to fall asleep. And despite seeming rather less vulnerable as they grow into toddlers and beyond, many nurslings are still in want of the breast most of the time, whether from habit or from need. When experiencing aversion, however, using breastfeeding as a kind of magic sleep tool becomes rather complicated. The restrictive situation of being stuck in a dark room, with a nursling physically attached to their breast and wholly dependent on her, can create a negative association with breastfeeding for the mother. With other factors, it is a pressure she cannot alleviate. And with no other way of getting her nursling to sleep, without massive crying outbursts and disruption to the family home, and often a siblings' environment too, she is stuck even if she no longer wants to continue a breastfeeding session. This can also be true for daytime contact naps (see the hashtag #contactnapping), but becomes particularly important at night. These are a few of what I term 'conditional breastfeeding' triggers for aversion:

1. Daytime dependency to fall asleep for naps.
2. Frequent requests for the breast/to breastfeed, often described as 'obsessive'.
3. The total length of time in a 24-hour period spent breastfeeding.
4. The length of time spent getting the nursling to sleep for naps or at bedtime.

When these conditional breastfeeding triggers are married to the touch and sensation triggers, you can see an instant relationship between them. Nipple twiddling, pinching, scratching and general incessant movement are all part of the breastfeeding experience, but how do they affect a mother when they happen on a very frequent basis, day and night? Is it true that the more you are pinched and scratched the more irritated you will become? When do things change from being 'annoying' to being triggers for aversion? Of course some folk do not experience aversion, and others are not bothered by the bodily antics, or do not have them happen so frequently, and for these mothers it may not be obvious why they might cause anger and rage. While pinching and scratching may happen in the newborn weeks as a baby's pincer reflex develops, we all know that if those teeny nails aren't clipped it can start to hurt as they frantically panic to latch. Now imagine these antics carrying on into toddlerhood, and it becomes a matter of preventing blood being drawn and visible cuts appearing on a mother's chest. Breastfeeding may not be a kinetic activity for *mothers*, but nurslings certainly move! All of their waking time. From babies to toddlers to children, movement is a fundamental and essential part of their social and biological development, and is an integral requirement for learning and growing. It is a necessity. A non-moving infant is always a cause for concern. As children get older movement becomes more controlled, more determined, and they become stronger – and breastfeeding mothers know this, as they are climbed on with the precision of a heat-seeking missile when their nurslings request feeds.

Although we understand the importance of the motor neuron development that happens through movement in nurslings, I would say we also have to consider the mother's tolerance level for this movement, and the reaction it can elicit as nurslings grow. If you are persistently tense when a certain kind of movement happens when you are breastfeeding, this will add to the vicious cycle of aversion, as it will act as a trigger. Nipple tweaking or twiddling is a case in point, and a common occurrence as well as a common trigger. There is a case to be made that this nipple twiddling encourages milk let-down, which I wouldn't ordinarily contest, but mothers with aversion who are clearly in discomfort and stressed by the activity of their nursling will be flooded with stress hormones that directly inhibit oxytocin, the hormone responsible for the let-down. So I would argue that nipple stimulation for the let-down at this point becomes futile, making it counterproductive for both mother and nursling. Consistently holding a nursling's hand from early on, preventing access to the other nipple and perhaps even any skin, is a good idea for mothers who struggle with a particular type of skin or nipple contact. What personally causes your aversion as a reaction to these triggers may vary, because one mother's trigger will not be the same as another's. Whether it is mole picking, ear twiddling, armpit digging, or that they are latched on all night when you are not someone who can sleep with constant bodily contact, these behaviours have different effects on different mothers. Frequent night feeds are well tolerated by some mothers, while others cannot cope because they take longer to get back to sleep after being awake breastfeeding at night. Some triggers won't apply because some mothers may be able to get their nurslings to sleep without breastfeeding, or only breastfeeding for two minutes. So it is not just about the possible triggers, but also the consideration that mothers often have sole responsibility for caring and the need for respite from this, both mentally and physically.

The real difficulty with this responsibility is that the responsiveness required to fulfil it does not stop at night. Being 'in service' as mothers who have nurtured through breastfeeding and have formed skinship bonds by taking care of nurslings at night as well as through the day, often means mothers have put their nurslings' needs before their own. This can, over time, cause great suffering and in some situations even pain for mothers, and this is not to be overlooked. It takes great strength to be a night-caring mother, while also being a day-caring mother, especially when the responsibility weighs on you alone. It is a strength that, arguably, some do not possess. It's no secret that I support mothers who cannot do it, who crack at the seams early on, and it often only becomes worse as time goes by. Single mothers, mothers without family or friend support, mothers who have a disability, mothers who are struggling with severe depression, stay-at-home mothers, mothers of multiples, mothers of nurslings with severe allergies . . . it all amounts to a sort of self-sacrifice, because caregiving takes up so much time and energy, and much of it is simply breastfeeding. I'd argue that this type of responsive-parenting sacrifice is something that some mothers cannot give for long lengths of time, which is perhaps one reason why we see a prevalence of sleep training. Of course there are many other confounding and contributing reasons why parents leave babies or toddlers to cry to sleep alone, including prevalent societal norms, unrealistic expectations of infant sleep behaviours and, crucially, the pressures of modernity with mothers needing to return to work. However, just *not being able to* physically, mentally, and emotionally cope with continuous responsive caregiving, night and day, is enough of a reason for mothers to opt for sleep training. And similarly, it is enough of a reason to trigger the onset of aversion, when the personal needs of a mother conflict with the requests of her nursling.

Nursling temperament and character

Aversion can be, in part, an experience that occurs when there is a clash between infant temperament and character and a breastfeeding mother's needs or preferences. Nurslings who need to be constantly held in the fourth trimester and who breastfeed often, sleep little, and need consistent connection and interaction (who will otherwise continuously cry) are necessarily more demanding of a mother's energy and time. This means that the chances of friction and conflict increase as time passes, and the mother's ability to meet her child's needs wanes. This conflict can manifest with symptoms of aversion if the mother feels the suffocation of conditional breastfeeds and has touch preference sensitivities, as the activity of breastfeeding will invariably trigger a reaction. Similarly, breastfeeding a boisterous older nursling who moves incessantly, is loud, rough in their body contact and often asks to feed is not the same experience as breastfeeding a gentler, timid and quiet nursling who is not too bothered about breastfeeding as they get older and start solids. I am not saying that aversion only occurs in the former case, just that it seems less likely to happen in the latter, at least not for the reason of nursling temperament and character alone, but rather for other reasons such as breastfeeding through pregnancy or due to persistent pain.

Individual preferences, individual limits in individual situations

Conclusively (or perhaps not so conclusively), mother and infant preference, temperament, character, dependency, pain and skin sensitivity, and home life play a role in triggers of aversion. Feeling 'touched out', with what seems like constant bodily contact, is a widely understood trigger. Crucially, what qualifies as 'constant' bodily contact may vary from mother to mother. A stay-at-home mother may have reached her limit after a total of nine hours of bodily contact a day. A picture of this day would include frequent night wakes and latching every couple of hours, after already spending two hours breastfeeding to get her nursling to sleep, a full 4–6am breastfeed in bed to keep her nursling asleep, and intermittent breastfeeds after breakfast that total 45 minutes. Add to that an hour-long breastfeeding session for a contact nap after lunch, more intermittent breastfeeding during the afternoon along with a couple of 20-minute breastfeeds after an emotional outburst or 'tantrum' (I don't like that word much, but hey). The final blow is another two-hour bedtime of on-off-on-off breastfeeding in order to get them to sleep, thinking that each time they latch back on that 'this time will do the trick'. This kind of typical day does not even account for increased breastfeeding time during frequent periods of teething, illness or developmental leaps.

A different picture would be of a full-time working mother who has been dealing with colleagues and deadlines all day, who just wants some time alone but has to sit down to breastfeed for a couple of hours to 'reconnect' with her nursling as soon as she walks in the door. All the time she is thinking of the million and one things she has to do for the next day but cannot as she is unable to get up – remember breastfeeding is rarely a kinetic activity for the mother as nurslings grow. In the first situation the actual time spent breastfeeding is a very large proportion of a 24-hour day, and in the second the time spent feeding was only a fraction in comparison. Nonetheless, the notion of feeling 'touched out' manifests in both scenarios. And both scenarios demonstrate that it takes extraordinary patience to be able to responsively parent and breastfeed on demand. You can reasonably see how an urge to de-latch and get up or stop breastfeeding may occur.

Urge to de-latch

Given our discussion of triggers, and what we know about the phenomenon of aversion, the overwhelming urge to de-latch is perhaps unsurprising. If you are feeling 'touched out' and you do not want to be touched, you will want to do something to stop being touched. If you are feeling anger, agitation or are irritated when doing a specific activity, it is only human to want to move away from it. Wouldn't you say this is a sane response? If something is uncomfortable for you, you want it to change so it becomes comfortable; if something is painful, you will want to stop the pain. De-latching nurslings achieves all of these goals and brings instant relief. And if you feel like a prisoner stuck in a dark room, you will want to re-claim your freedom and exercise your autonomy over your body. If you feel trapped because of having to sit down and breastfeed for hours, or you have to cook or work or are bursting for the loo, you will want to stop breastfeeding and go cook or work or go to the loo. It's not rocket science. Yet a breastfeeding mother who is a responsive-parent, and parenting alone, is more restricted when it comes to personal autonomy, including in freedom of movement and the ability to meet her own needs for self-care. I am not saying that breastfeeding actually makes you a prisoner, or means you have little bodily autonomy, just that it is the case that some women *feel* as though they are trapped, or that they have little control over their body. When some mothers with aversion post about feeling violated or used, it doesn't mean they think their nursling is actually violating them or abusing them, but that they *feel* like this at the time. It can be a frequent, perhaps truer feeling, for mothers who are survivors of previous sexual abuse. A whole array of mixed emotions and challenges come up for these mothers when breastfeeding, and it is common for women who have been abused to post in the aversion support groups.

Triggers that are related to past trauma or anything that causes significant stress, whether conscious or unconscious, are important in the vicious cycle of aversion. This is due to the fact that if there is any *perceived* threat by a mother, particularly at night, even if it isn't real, the fight or flight stress response will kick in before she knows it. Breastfeeding itself can trigger very real memories from previous sexual abuse. Negative feelings may overwhelm you on a purely biological level as adrenalin floods your system and the parasympathetic nervous system is activated: your mind will scream at you to 'de-latch and runaway'. The situation has become a matter of self-preservation, which explains the *urge* mothers describe with aversion. As many psychologists will attest, it is difficult for your body not to do what your mind tells it to when there is a perceived threat. In fact, the adrenalin that is released is there precisely in order to get you ready to act, to move, to protect yourself. The urge to de-latch can be difficult to contain for some women, and can mean that there are incidents of 'premature' de-latching. By this I mainly mean before the *nursling* is ready, or has de-latched of their own accord. The exact amount of time needed to breastfeed can't be specified, as it can vary from nursling to nursling depending on the circumstances. Premature de-latching, especially if it is not done in a gentle, loving way, may leave the nursling feeling upset. If the nursling is gently de-latched but isn't distracted instantly they may still want to breastfeed, so they may ask to breastfeed again, or cry uncontrollably and need to be consoled, leading a responsive mother to breastfeed again depending on when she 'gives in'. Offering a hug or kisses just will not cut it for some nurslings. It will make the situation worse, because you are refusing the breast that they are indicating they need. Stress levels rise for both mother and nursling. The vicious cycle places the breastfeeding mother in a compromised position, as aversion will likely strike again in this situation. Thus the cycle continues, and the mother is powerless to stop it without her letting her nursling cry persistently, which can affect family life as well as her emotions. Some nurslings will accept reductions and limitations on access to the breast, while others categorically will not. The phrase 'stuck between a rock and a hard place' has never felt so true for a mother stuck in this vicious cycle day in day out, night in and night out. Sending a clear, consistent message would bring some order and balance, and stop the vicious cycle, but this means either continuing to breastfeed on demand without de-latching, or stopping breastfeeding altogether. And for mothers with aversion, both those options are fraught with an array of difficulties and negative feelings. To continue to breastfeed with aversion means being frustrated, agitated, angry, trapped, used, stuck and acting like a mother you do not recognise. Stopping breastfeeding means feelings of sadness, loss, selfishness, failure, weakness, and even causing harm to the nursling you love: again, acting like a mother you do not recognise as yourself.

The guilt, the shame, and the will

Distress about having to breastfeed, not wanting to breastfeed, hating breastfeeding or just the thought of having to sit through the next breastfeeding session is common in mothers who experience aversion. Guilt in every one of those scenarios also applies: about not enjoying breastfeeding, about projecting the negative feelings onto their nursling and about de-latching or deterring their nursling and having to deal with the consequences. The guilt about not enjoying breastfeeding is coupled with concern about not having the 'normal' feelings that a mother 'should':

> *I've had a few incidents of aversion but it only happens at night. I get severe restless legs and my whole body feels like it's just rejecting breastfeeding. I end up begging my husband to get them off me as I shout 'what is wrong with me?' Then I cry, and have to leave the room. I feel so guilty and upset, I love feeding my boys and I love them.* Karen, Peru

Aversion and subsequent guilt are often followed by shame. It is the projection of negative feelings onto the nursling when breastfeeding that causes shame, along with the notion that negative feelings when breastfeeding are abnormal and you are a bad mother for feeling them. A loving, responsive mother who, with aversion, suddenly changes her temperament is not a comfortable self-image. There is a sense of emotional turmoil that increases with the frequency or severity of aversion (and the subsequent conflict that can arise). This emotional burden can be triggered repeatedly and continues throughout the day and night if aversion is persistent, and it can become a source of deep and often lasting upset. Aversion becomes a source of internal conflict within the mother's mind and heart because she cannot breastfeed with ease, but cannot wean with ease either. Aversion is also a source of external conflict that spills over into home life, especially if there is frequent premature de-latching, or attempts to wean. And if you are a mother who does not know about aversion, it can be incredibly confusing to start getting these feelings. The guilt and the shame that arise are there because of a sort of deep need to nurture, and the invisible importance of skinship, which, with the symptoms of aversion, means breastfeeding starts to become the problem, not the solution.

Internal conflict and confusion

The internal conflict and anguish of aversion is often spoken about in support groups, as mothers feel anger and agitation, the overwhelming urge to de-latch or remove their nursling, while at the *same time* wanting to be able to protect, hold, nurture and basically *breastfeed them*. But they can't.

> *(It) first happened when he was just a couple of months old. I felt like I had been put in the middle of a storm, I had an energy inside me that made me feel like I wanted to scream or hit things. I was feeding at the time, I said to my fiancé 'I feel like I don't want him feeding!' But of course, I felt awful for feeling like that. All I wanted was to hold and nourish him.*
> Rosanna, Hong Kong

Our biological instinct as mothers – which is regulated, supported and reinforced by oxytocin – is to protect our offspring; the experience of aversion is the manifestation of precisely the opposite of this instinct. I wanted to know why this happens. We all (mothers with aversion) want to know why it happens. Another key question I wanted to answer was why mothers continue to breastfeed when they experience aversion. I believe the answers lie, in part at least, in the role of oxytocin. Oxytocin released when breastfeeding creates the unseen connection mothers have to their nurslings; a bond that is considered strong and lifelong. It is not easy to break, hence both mother and nursling's reluctance to cease breastfeeding entirely. But the stress response that seems to be triggered when aversion strikes means that we also have a sort of negative, misplaced use of the oxytocin that is released in the body; a fight or flight state when a mother is breastfeeding. And this is not the only possible biological cause of aversion.

PART III

The Pleasure
and The Pain

5

It's Just Biology

And yet the body in extremis – the body experiencing itself acutely as a body – is a human reality to which mothers cannot help but have access, although once again they are expected to put a lid on it, to make everything sweet and nice. They can, they must, love, hold, cuddle their babies, but on condition of warding off the danger of any spillages – blood, guts, misery and lust. Their task is to prevent such intensities from going too far, to clean out the drains, on behalf of everyone.*

Becoming a mother, much like becoming an adolescent, is full of all kinds of changes, biological and emotional. In fact, one paper in the early 1970s called for the word 'matrescence' to describe the whole transformation that takes place from conception to birth to motherhood, because it really is monumental and needs its own word.** When I read the paper, I began to wonder: is it the breastfeeding or is it the responsive parenting required in motherhood that is driving mothers to feel the way they do and get aversion? Often, mothers find their nursling or nurslings intense; or rather, they need a lot of contact and a lot of comforting that is very full-on. If responsive mothers are not breastfeeding, they are cuddling or baby-wearing; always doing something together, always sharing personal space. And supposedly, thereby, creating

---

*   Rose, J. (2018). *Mothers: An Essay on Love and Cruelty* (Main edition). London: Faber & Faber, p62.

**   Matrescence. *Education, Theory & Practice.* (n.d.). Retrieved 25 October 2019 www.matrescence.com

the peaceful state of *anshin* that come from skinship in the family home, and by extension in their own selves. So, are these aspects of motherhood making mothers feel worn down and 'touched out', or is it the activity of breastfeeding alone? Is it motherhood that makes women feel as though they are losing ownership of their body, or is it the act of breastfeeding that is responsible the for feelings of loss of control and lack of consent that can lead to negative emotions? I would argue it is both, and that it is not an either/or situation. Mothers who breastfeed are in a *breastfeeding motherhood*: breastfeeding and motherhood are intertwined, irreversibly interlinked and often inseparable. And although aversion is triggered for a number of reasons that can differ from mother to mother, these can still be categorised and have clear causal patterns attributed to them. They have physiological or psychological mechanisms, and often a combination of both. The problem then is not that aversion exists as an experience in a breastfeeding mother, but that it is somehow considered by society as abnormal or even morally wrong, when in fact for many women it is simply a result of biology.

Hidden biology

The explosion of honest and empowering posts by mothers on social media is, I feel, a movement that is a reaction to the wholly hidden, perhaps even oppressed, human side of what being a mother entails. Experiential outpours and the graphic, real-time images of birth, breastfeeding and the struggles of mothers have meant there is another narrative emerging to counter the idealism of motherhood that has prevailed in the last few centuries. What motherhood is *really like*, how much you can struggle and suffer to your utter core, and how much it can be hated at times is now an accessible alternative story that mothers are sharing. But the thing is, you only seem to have access to this narrative once you've already gone through the darkness or, if you are lucky, are stuck in the thick of it and have found a post or pages that raise awareness of the 'realness' of motherhood. Remember most social media accounts won't be spending millions of pounds on advertising like companies that promote idealised versions of mothering. It's more likely we will see adverts and perfect images portraying what it is to be a perfect mother, with a perfect baby, than the dreary monotonousness of motherhood or the raw darkness it can bring out. Which leaves us at risk of normalising the former, unbeknownst to us, on a subconscious level – because that is how advertising works, after all. We have, most of us, gone through life and not been taught anything about the process of birth, the biology of lactation, or the basics of breastfeeding. We have also, at least in affluent countries with big public and population-level health promotion campaigns, been told that breast is best and breastfeeding is the right thing to do. Before becoming mothers, that is about all we really knew. So when breastfeeding difficulties happen, mothers without appropriate and educated people to support them will not be able to continue breastfeeding unless they have a strong will of their own. It is the will of the mother, that stubborn determination, that is the driving force. And at least on one level the same applies when aversion strikes: without strong determination on the mother's part, the breastfeeding relationship will likely come to an end. We currently do not know how many women just stop breastfeeding when they start to get aversion. We do not know how common it is, and therefore we cannot know how 'normal' it is.

I think that making sense of aversion is understanding that it is a part of the breastfeeding journey for some mothers. We don't know about it because we have not been exposed to it, because of how motherhood has been portrayed, and because women have been generally shunned into silence while being moulded into each culture's version of the Stepford housewife. Aversion simply doesn't fit into the prevalent picture of a 'good mother', not only for others and society, but for the mothers themselves. As a mother, you don't see yourself as a tetchy, angry person who cannot bear to be touched by your child. It is confusing, upsetting and disorientating. Even those with a strong determination to continue breastfeeding soon tire of the negative emotions and having the urge to take their nursling off their breast – but this doesn't mean they want to stop breastfeeding, as we have seen. As responsive, loving mothers, we see ourselves as *breastfeeding mothers*, continuing the dynamic that was often established from the newborn days: the baby asks, we give. It seems on one level quite bizarre to experience aversion. And so the oft-repeated question is asked: 'Why am I getting aversion?'

There is sometimes, but not always, a simple answer. Aversion can occur and is the *start* of the weaning process for many mothers of older nurslings – in the mammalian world we see quite shocking examples of maternal aggression when weaning off mother's milk. If this response is normal for those animals, then perhaps it is normal for some of us – lest we forget: we are mammals too. If you have your menses while breastfeeding, hormones around this time can make you agitated, while also making your breasts sore and nipples sensitive. This, naturally, results in mothers not wanting to breastfeed or finding it more difficult. When these biological changes are added to the array of personal triggers we have previously covered – your child's temperament and needs, and the feelings of being 'touched out' – it seems clear why aversion may arise in these breastfeeding mothers. When the reasons for aversion are not clear, it becomes more of a layering exercise, as the simple reasons make way for the complex. In exploring this, I will show how aversion can be multifactorial and biopsychosocial in nature.[*]

Before beginning, I want to point out something that often isn't acknowledged, which is that being pregnant, lactating, carrying and caring for infants adds up to a considerable energetic cost for women.[**] This cost is cumulatively substantial when you consider that there can be repeated cycles over many years of some women's lives. Picciano estimates the combined caloric cost of gestation and breastfeeding to be 200,000

---

[*]   There is often an interplay of physiological, psychological and social factors at play when mothers struggle, and aversion is no exception.

[**] See Jasienka 2009 & Prentice *et al* 1996, on pg 171 in Tomori, C., E. L. Palmquist, A., & Quinn, E. A. (Eds.). (2017). *Breastfeeding* (1st edition). Milton Park, Abingdon, Oxon; New York, NY: Routledge.

calories.* Although this acknowledges that there are some 'costs' when making little humans, calculating it purely in calories does not help us to understand other, more 'invisible' costs: for example the cumulative mental health costs of being a primary caregiver, or the costs of the impact of modern-day stress on the job of mothering. How calorific and mental health costs, and the inevitable depletion of a mother's ability to meet these costs over time, will vary from mother to mother, both in terms of her sociodemographic status and subsequent support network, and also her bodily biology, because these are all linked and there is always an interplay. It would be both unfair and naive to think that this 'energetic' cost expenditure does not affect a mother's experience of breastfeeding, and so her character and emotions *while* breastfeeding. Even though the overwhelming majority of women can *make* milk, breastfeeding is not just the making of milk: it is the will to establish a supply, the activity of feeding, the sustaining of life, the sacrifice of sleep, the restriction of her life, and the mental, emotional and physical burden of it all. It is, for those who *mother through breastfeeding*, a substantial and incalculable cost of nurturing a small human. A priceless gift.

The point at which a mother can no longer sustain the considerable and often very intensive breastfeeding costs, in terms of energy and time expenditure, will be the point at which the weaning process kicks in from her side.** For some women, it may not always be a 'true' cost that is causing her to stop breastfeeding, but a severe lack of support, or lack of respite, and the burden of the perceived cost of breastfeeding because of this. You can be frustrated about spending 45 minutes breastfeeding to sleep, but until you stop breastfeeding to sleep, you are never going to know how difficult it can be to get an infant to sleep without the breast! In some ways,

---

*   See Picannio, 2003 on p172 in Tomori, C., E. L. Palmquist, A., & Quinn, E. A. (Eds.). (2017). *Breastfeeding* (1st edition). Milton Park, Abingdon, Oxon; New York, NY: Routledge.
** See economic trade offs in Tomori, C., E. L. Palmquist, A., & Quinn, E. A. (Eds.). (2017). *Breastfeeding* (1st edition). Milton Park, Abingdon, Oxon; New York, NY: Routledge.

it is easy to blame challenging aspects of mothering on breastfeeding when it becomes difficult or we do not want to do it. But stopping breastfeeding isn't always the answer to our problems, even if the problem is aversion. The crucial thing for most women who get aversion is to decipher whether the aversion is a true biological trigger for weaning, or whether it is the body's response to a biological, personal, family, social or work difficulty that is adding further stress to the mother's already full time job of breastfeeding, and what this is 'costing' her. With aversion, how do we know when to change the situation by weaning, or when to improve the breastfeeding set up, or address a mother's thought processes? And when is it simply a matter of biology, and her body just saying 'no' to breastfeeding at that time? It turns out there are some very clear ways of knowing, starting with ovulation, menstruation and pregnancy.

Ovulation

Some women can correlate their experience of aversion to the start of their 'green week' every month, even pinpointing it to ovulation (tracking your menstrual cycles with an app makes this possible), so their aversion could be etiologically hormonal. Recently, I read that testosterone peaks in women when they ovulate. Testosterone, it seems, is not only found in men, as we were taught in biology 101. This is not hugely surprising, as both sexes can be prone to aggression or violence, and conversely both are able to show compassionate behaviour and secure bonding, which is attributed to testosterone's antagonist, oxytocin. Testosterone is mainly known for the typically male tendencies of aggression and motivation for sex, because it is found in higher concentration in men. So how is this related to aversion? Well, testosterone actually prevents the binding of oxytocin to its receptors, so that the calm and loving state that breastfeeding can evoke is directly inhibited. If you get aversion when you ovulate, and you don't feel as responsive and caring toward your nursling, testosterone can explain why you feel like that. Biologically, this peak in testosterone can make you feel a little 'on heat' too, thereby seeking out a partner for sex – great timing with your body releasing an egg. But sex is not usually on the agenda for mothers who responsively breastfeed on demand day and night and who are consequently 'touched out' as it is. Knowing you are ovulating, and observing the changes in your mood and propensity for frustration and aggression, can help ride out the couple of days it lasts.

Menstruation

Premenstrual tension and post-menstrual tension is experienced by many menstruating women and although it doesn't always plague their lives, for some women it can be crippling. If your menses return while breastfeeding, you may also get the return of menstrual tension. Lots of women feel a lot more irritated during and after their period when their oestrogen levels are low and progesterone naturally dips, which affects chemicals in the brain.* Getting your period can certainly affect your breastfeeding ability and even your relationship with your nursling. Different hormones than the rest of the cycle are rife and the body drastically changes – with the increasing size of the womb and tenderness of the breasts – all making breastfeeding uncomfortable. Being stuck in an activity that is uncomfortable is likely to make doing it harder, and when you are committed to it – as you usually are when breastfeeding – this creates an additional tension and pressure. Many women have the feeling that everything is 'just off' when they are menstruating, and along with the tension that builds during this time, shielding your nursling from aversion when you are trying to manage the changes in your body can become that bit harder. Under pressure, people can become agitated and angry, especially when they have no way out. You can't explain to your eight-month-old that you have your period and don't want to breastfeed today because it's uncomfortable! It doesn't work

---

* Yonkers, K. A., O'Brien, P. M. S., & Eriksson, E. (2008). Premenstrual syndrome. *Lancet*, *371*(9619), 1200–1210.

like that with breastfeeding. It doesn't work like that with responsive parenting in the early months.

Pregnancy

The changes that happen while carrying a little human are hugely different to your normal body activity as a woman. While some of us can effortlessly pull it off, others are not so lucky and are rendered incapable of getting out of bed when pregnant. Pregnancy can affect your breastfeeding ability and experience, depending on where you fall on the spectrum of how much being pregnant affects your body and breasts. According to Newton and Theotokatos, who conducted a study with 503 breastfeeding women, the majority reported breast soreness and nipple sensitivity, alongside discomfort and pain when breastfeeding through pregnancy.[*] Hormones play such a large role in the body's changes, and hormones have very complex relationships. The differing role of progesterone is a good case in point here. Milk production during pregnancy is lessened for some mothers, as it is inhibited by placental hormones like progesterone. And although up to 70% of women noticed a reduction in milk, only around 18% reported that it dried up completely.[**] A drop in supply is notoriously noticed by nurslings, who tend to nurse more and fidget more to stimulate the let-down. Both of these can mean that aversion strikes, and if the milk does 'dry up' and a nursling dry-nurses, this too can cause discomfort for a mother. Weaning is common at this point, but doesn't always happen as many mothers and nurslings are not yet ready to wean entirely off the breast – so continuing to breastfeed until birth of the newborn is not uncommon. Later on in the pregnancy progesterone decreases, and this is correlated with an increase in milk volume in the first days after birth. This may be why the mothers who have made it

---

[*]   Newton, N., & Theotokatos, M. (1979). Breast-feeding during pregnancy in 503 women: Does a psychobiological weaning mechanism exist in humans? *In Emotion and Reproduction.*

[**] Moscone, S. R., & Moore, M. J. (1993). Breastfeeding during pregnancy. *Journal of Human Lactation: Official Journal of International Lactation Consultant Association,* 9(2), 83–88.

through pregnancy with aversion suddenly see it disappear with the arrival of the baby and the milk. Perhaps more oxytocin has an effect too, because of more frequent let-downs.

Breastfeeding through such extreme body changes is no mean feat, as changes in size and sensitivity of the chest area and tummy mean adapting the positioning of a nursling's suckling to try to maximise comfort – often to no avail. And then we must take into account the energetic cost of lactating, the struggle with building skinship through breastfeeding, and maintaining the dynamics of nurturing and responsive mothering through breastfeeding:

> *When I was pregnant I was sure my milk supply was less, but he seemed to want to breastfeed more. The pain was almost unbearable, I don't know how I carried on, but I had always fed on demand and it was just the way we did things. I couldn't just stop. My aversion was mild when he was a toddler, but when I became pregnant it became severe. It plagued our lives.* Alisha, Ottawa

Pain, persistent pain and discomfort

When I heard Dr Kristin Tully speak at a lactation conference years ago, one sentence that stuck in my head was that 'breastfeeding is time consuming, can be painful and some women encounter comments which can be undermining'*. Perhaps it was because I was relatively new to the field, or because I had only been a breastfeeding mother for a few years with only one nursling, but this was the first time I had actually heard someone say anything that acknowledged what I was going through. Back then, in my non-academic world of friends who were breastfeeding mothers, breastfeeding was not often spoken about as 'time consuming', and as for pain, the only thing I was told repeatedly is that 'breastfeeding shouldn't be painful'. But of course the reality is that it simply is painful

---

*   Kristin Tully, PhD, "*Understanding and supporting early postpartum maternal mental health needs*", iLactation conference lectures, 2017: ilactation.com/conferences/our-10th-conference/

for some mothers. It can be very painful, and persistently so.

According to the International Association for the Study of Pain, pain is defined as an unpleasant sensory and emotional experience associated with actual or potential tissue damage.* It is possible in the early days of breastfeeding that women can experience *acute* pain, which is when pain is provoked by something specific, and only occurs for a short period of time. Engorgement from milk coming in, your nipples hardening as they get accustomed to feeding, or soreness from an inadequate or improper latch are all common reasons. But one study by McCann *et al* found that 38% of breastfeeding women experienced persistent sore nipples, even after the early days had long since passed. In the paper they described the confusion and surprise of these women, as well as the intensity and duration of the pain; women even used the words 'excruciating' and 'horrific'. If we think of a normal human response to pain, the symptoms of aversion like the 'urge to de-latch' and intrusive thoughts of 'throwing the child off' and 'running away' seem reasonable. In fact, I would argue they are biologically natural, because this kind of acute pain is also associated with the sympathetic nervous system or the 'fight or flight' response kicking in. Your heart rate increases, you have a rush of adrenaline to help you take action and the urge to move (presumably to safety). This is not very helpful for a breastfeeding mother, in a dark room at night, unable to move because you are breastfeeding a nursling and desperate for them to sleep so you can too. Where does that adrenaline go? While this fight or flight system served a useful biological purpose of getting us out of danger when at risk of being mauled by a bear in our cavewomen days, it is not so useful in the 21st century. And even less so when it comes to mothers who are triggered to get aversion through pain. Pain is actually a part of breastfeeding in many ways. You cannot say it doesn't exist, both in the short term, and for longer periods of time for some mothers. Breastfeeding difficulties like poor latch, blocked ducts, infections, milk blebs and even the

---

*   Treede R. D. (2018). The International Association for the Study of Pain definition of pain: as valid in 2018 as in 1979, but in need of regularly updated footnotes. *Pain reports*, 3(2), e643.

nurslings themselves can cause pain: McClellan *et al* published a study that showed some infants had a higher vacuuming suction than others, which mothers found painful.* We don't know much about individual genetic polymorphisms related to pain sensitivity in breastfeeding mothers, but we know enough to understand it can affect the breastfeeding experience for some women.** People have different thresholds for pain, it's related to your genes, and because of this people have different skin sensitivities.

There are several other causes of breast and nipple pain in the early days, but mothers can experience these alongside *lasting* pain that is often found in those who have nurslings with feed-inhibiting tongue-ties, or have infections like thrush, or experience vasospasm*** – and these are certainly not uncommon in the aversion community. As well as this kind of fight or flight response with aversion, you can also see a slow kind of avoidance of breastfeeding set in with these mothers. This is when they start exhibit avoidant behaviour due to persistent pain, known as *chronic* pain, which is when pain generally lasts beyond the body's usual healing times. Whether it is a gradual onset of pain, or pain that doesn't go away, some women have unexplained pain:

> *When I went to the doctor they said the infection had gone and the nipple had healed from when it had a lesion. They could find nothing wrong in the way he was feeding, and they checked my breasts and saw nothing wrong, but it was so painful to feed. I don't care if they couldn't see anything, I know what pain feels like.* Betty, Calgary

---

* McClellan, H., Geddes, D., Kent, J., Garbin, C., Mitoulas, L., & Hartmann, P. (2008). Infants of mothers with persistent nipple pain exert strong sucking vacuums. Acta paediatrica (Oslo, Norway: 1992), 97(9), 1205–1209. https://doi.org/10.1111/j.1651-2227.2008.00882.x.

** Lucas, R., Bernier, K., Perry, M., Evans, H., Ramesh, D., Young, E., ... Starkweather, A. (2019). Promoting self-management of breast and nipple pain in breastfeeding women: Protocol of a pilot randomized controlled trial. *Research in Nursing & Health, 42*(3), 176–188.

*** Buck, M. L., Amir, L. H., Cullinane, M., & Donath, S. M. (2013). Nipple Pain, Damage, and Vasospasm in the First 8 Weeks Postpartum. *Breastfeeding Medicine, 9*(2), 56–62.

Experiencing pain even after visible physical damage is gone, and the body looks healed, is a phenomenon that occurs. So, why is there persistent pain? In the pain literature there is a model of pain-fear avoidance that describes how people can develop musculoskeletal pain as a result of avoidant behaviours that are based on their fears. Are the negative emotions of aversion and the intrusive thoughts due to pain-fear avoidance for some women? A manifestation of their fear of being harmed, fear of being trapped, fear of being in pain itself? Is there an associative expected pain that has been 'learned' over time with a mother who had struggled with breastfeeding and had ongoing pain in the early days? It is not unreasonable to think that a kind of 'sensitisation' is happening in these mothers. This is when someone responds to certain stimuli in a sensitive way. Normally associated with systemic changes, such as those in the nervous system, 'sensitisation' could be attributed to the dread that hits you before the next feed – one of the symptoms of aversion. Pain – whether visibly real, or experienced as real, it doesn't matter – the dread of feeling pain has a huge effect on mothers, as nipple pain and damage experienced in mothers is actually linked with other conditions like depression and anxiety,[*] and is a considerable challenge for women. It is clear that breastfeeding in the presence of persistent pain can and does affect your behaviour, and we know that what affects your behaviour affects your emotions.

If your aversion is manifesting due to pain, we have to know the characteristics of pain, and identify its cause to be able to understand what is going on, and what can help. A sudden onset of pain could be associated with a blocked duct, for example, or perhaps a damaged nipple, either from an infant biting it, or using the wrong size flange on a pump. There are changes that can be made and treatment options are available. If the pain is sporadic and you are not sure why you get it, it would be worthwhile keeping a diary or tracking your menstrual cycle, because we know hormones have a role to play in aversion. Even though menses themselves don't

---

[*]   Ibid.

necessarily last that long, the before and after effects can last at least a couple of weeks of every month for some women:

> *Before I fell pregnant I never really noticed changes in my breasts, sure they felt a bit sore around my period but that was it. When I had Alfie, I didn't expect my periods to return so soon, but at three months postpartum they were back, and it seemed like for ten days to two weeks of every month my breasts were sore, and my nipples were sensitive to contact. It made nursing him really tricky as it almost always irritated me in that time and I really had to stop myself from taking him off.* Bryanny, Perth

However, if the pain is persistent, there is probably something else that has been missed, like an undiagnosed or unsuccessfully treated tie, vasospasm or perhaps an unconscious response to trauma you have experienced. It would be worthwhile considering seeing a breastfeeding specialist to have a proper assessment, because if pain is the root cause of your aversion, then addressing this is the only way to address aversion for you and your nursling. There is also some scope in these three clear causes of persistent pain that you can self-identify.

Trauma, ties and vasospasm

The biological, psychological and social consequences of trauma in mothers are numerous and interconnected, with rates of post-traumatic stress disorder ranging from anywhere from 1–21% depending on the cohort studied, and up to 45% in high-risk samples.[*] We know that birth and breastfeeding are linked, both biologically with lactogenesis and also because of the impact of birth interventions and mode of delivery on breastfeeding. Trauma in mothers can happen at birth if there is obstetric violence (a recognised description of a particular

---

[*]   Khoramroudi, R. (2018). The prevalence of posttraumatic stress disorder during pregnancy and the postpartum period. *Journal of Family Medicine and Primary Care, 7*(1), 220–223.

kind of attack that can happen to women when giving birth, when they are vulnerable, ranging from being ignored to being told to 'shut up' during labour, having vaginal sweeps and synthetic oxytocin like Syntocinon or Pitocin without asking for it, and being pressured into having epidurals and other interventions without informed consent).* Birth is often a hugely traumatic event for many women, and research has shown this to affect breastfeeding, whether because of substances like drugs in the body affecting the baby's ability to latch, because of physical interventions affecting your or your baby's ability to breastfeed, or because of the shock of the birth and your response to the baby. Synthetic oxytocin is now used in hospital settings to speed up labour, but can mean labour is actually more painful. Having a perineal tear or having major abdominal surgery (otherwise known as a caesarean section) can mean a painful, less speedy recovery from the work of birth. If birth is not supported or it goes horribly wrong, then the experience is deeply traumatic. Trauma is such a key part of the story of aversion because of its impact on the lives of mothers postnatally, and how it sets the trajectory of a breastfeeding relationship. Starting a relationship with trauma is not always going to make it an easy relationship to be in, and the breastfeeding relationship is no exception, because trauma doesn't just 'go away'. Some experts claim our body holds on to trauma. It seeps out in the way we deal with things, the way we feel – and our bodies can even manifest it as pain, because even if trauma is psychological, it is a somatic experience. There are many studies to show that clear biological symptoms and conditions can arise after a traumatic experience.**

The connection isn't one way. When trauma itself is recognised, traditional understandings of pain mechanisms often lead pain to be attributed to some psychological disturbance – not just the physical or biological. Biological

---

* Jardim, D. M. B., & Modena, C. M. (2018). Obstetric violence in the daily routine of care and its characteristics. *Revista Latino-Americana de Enfermagem, 26.*

** McFarlane, A. C. (2010). The long-term costs of traumatic stress: Intertwined physical and psychological consequences. *World Psychiatry, 9*(1), 3–10.

conditions like vasospasm have actually been linked to emotional stress.* Vasospasm in the nipple is a reduced flow of blood through the capillaries which is caused by constriction in the circulation. For breastfeeding mothers who experience vasospasm, cold temperatures and poor latch can make feeding unbearably painful. Although vasospasm is known to be experienced by those who suffer with Raynaud's phenomenon, it is also linked to some medications used in pregnancy, breast surgery, and autoimmune diseases.** You may think, as I did for many years, that it was a purely physical condition, but a paper by Buck and colleagues suggests that vasospasm is not only due to the mechanical forces of the breastfeeding nursling, but that it is also associated with a combination of emotional and hormonal, as well as physiological, changes that come with childbirth.*** We cannot rule out the effects of the combination of trauma and pain in some mothers: their aversion is how their bodies respond to these difficulties. Even if you are dealing with a challenge that seems purely biological, like vasospasm or restrictive tongue-tie in your nursling, aversion can creep in as your body manifests the symptoms as a response to persistent pain or previous trauma.

Tongue-tie, or 'ankyloglossia', refers to a restriction of movement in an area under the tongue called the lingual frenulum. It is a normal anatomical structure and it is considered responsible for 'tongue-tie' in a small minority of infants as it has a role in the position of nerves in the area, and in stabilising tongue movement which is needed for optimal suckling. The knowledge, assessment, surgical revision and management of ties is not yet wholly understood and therefore not yet clinically valued (a bit like aversion!), yet time and again mothers in persistent pain in aversion support groups state that they are breastfeeding nurslings with tongue-ties. Like women who breastfeed through months of pregnancy, or with Raynaud's syndrome, or nipple damage, pain becomes

---

*   Buck, M. L., Amir, L. H., Cullinane, M., & Donath, S. M. (2013).
    Nipple Pain, Damage, and Vasospasm in the First 8 Weeks Postpartum. *Breastfeeding Medicine*, 9(2), 56–62.
** Ibid.
*** Ibid.

a regular part of their daily breastfeeding experience. Pain severity and pain tolerance is very complex and varies from person to person, but it is common to have negative emotions when in pain, and it is therefore not unexpected that the symptoms of aversion occur in women with breastfeeding journeys that are persistently painful. Interestingly, new research has suggested that negative emotions like anger and sadness can actually *cause* pain, as well as being a result of it.* This may add to our understanding of why some women with aversion experience persistent pain when breastfeeding even if there is no visible reason for it. If emotions from pain function as stressors,** and pain itself functions as a stressor, inflammation overall can be promoted in the body and we see another layer in the vicious cycle of aversion shown in Figure 3 (see page 36). You would have to be dosed up on a strong painkiller like morphine not to react to pain when breastfeeding, and not to have an urge to de-latch!

We may have established that trauma and pain are linked, that moving away from pain is normal, and that symptoms of aversion for mothers who experience pain are a reasonable response, but what is less clear is why mothers continue to breastfeed. One key finding from my researching this book, from supporting other women and from my own personal experience, is that time and again women continue to breastfeed despite experiencing aversion. There are a few factors at play to answer this question: not only is there a consideration of the strong bond oxytocin creates, but mothers also have their own personal goals and expectations that play into their motivations to continue breastfeeding, despite challenges. Then there is nursling conflict, and the reluctance to reduce or stop breastfeeding which also plays a large role:

---

*   Graham-Engeland, J. E., Song, S., Mathur, A., Wagstaff, D. A., Klein, L. C., Whetzel, C., & Ayoub, W. T. (2018). Emotional State Can Affect Inflammatory Responses to Pain Among Rheumatoid Arthritis Patients: Preliminary Findings. *Psychological Reports*, 33294118796655.

**   Lumley, M. A., Cohen, J. L., Borszcz, G. S., Cano, A., Radcliffe, A. M., Porter, L. S., … Keefe, F. J. (2011). Pain and Emotion: A Biopsychosocial Review of Recent Research. *Journal of Clinical Psychology*, 67(9), 942–968.

F was born prematurely, I can't describe how hard the first few months of his life were, and how hard I worked to establish my supply and get him to latch. Those days were dark but I never experienced aversion. It was only when he was much older, around 18 months, when it hit, and it was so hard to breastfeed but I had such an ordeal to have this special relationship I really didn't want to just stop. Besides, any attempts to cut feeds out of our day and night weren't taken very well by him. He just would not accept no for an answer! Laura, Warwick

When considering breastfeeding within the larger picture of a mother's daily life, it becomes clear that the mother has other confounding factors to weigh up. Some of these reasons we have covered, like mothers knowing a lot about the benefits of their tailored breastmilk for their nurslings. Who doesn't want the best for their child? For those with nurslings under the age of 12 months, knowing that milk is the main source of nutrition for the first year can mean they want to continue and not offer formula. The already established skinship relationship for mothers, particularly who bed-share, and the inextricable link to breastfeeding as a night-time practice, is a big deciding factor. And then there is the (often very emotionally charged) response of a prematurely de-latched nursling, or one who is refused the breast, and the sheer chaos that it can bring into the family home, especially at night. This means a mother will simply carry on breastfeeding. Emotions from both parties count in a breastfeeding relationship and can make a situation where aversion is experienced quite emotionally volatile. In reality, the bottom line is that it is not as simple as just 'stopping' breastfeeding in that moment, and even less simple to just 'stop' breastfeeding all together. People who have not experienced this kind of daily dilemma around refusing the breast due to being in pain or discomfort will probably be surprised when they find out you are still breastfeeding, and especially if you get aversion. Actually, a great many mothers themselves do not understand why they continue to breastfeed despite pain, and despite aversion. I think part of this surprise could be attributed to the fact that we don't place great importance on the very intricate and intimate nature of breastfeeding. It's not just the milk, it is everything else. It is *emotional milk* linked to our very core as a mother, and with the concepts of skinship and nurture, we understand that it is a way of life. And besides, breastfeeding involves two or more parties, one of which is experiencing the pain, for example, and the other which either cannot or does not understand this.* How can a mother move away from breastfeeding because of pain when she knows a nursling cannot understand her pain, and she knows it's not her nursling's fault? Tully and Ball found that most women report both positive and negative feelings about breastfeeding, and that mothers are continually balancing trade-offs that translate into factors affecting their perseverance in breastfeeding.** Breastfeeding, much like birth, involves very complex interactions for mothers. This means, in short, that one cannot simply *move away* from breastfeeding, even if it is painful.***.**** The complexity of the decision-making involved when there is the additional consideration of the nursling's needs is one clear reason why some mothers continue, such as nursling allergies or food intolerance for example. Another is that bonding that has developed through skinship and breastfeeding is very strong, and although the positive and pleasant aspects of this bonding can slowly slip away as the vicious cycle of aversion and de-latching continues with the increase in negative emotional turmoil, the bond remains. The strength of this bond, facilitated primarily by oxytocin, is a formidable and primal link, forged into the very core of our mothering. Understanding oxytocin's role in attachment helps

---

* The ability to empathise in a way that would mean a nursling would give up their breastfeeding session would not be possible until they are cognitively able to, generally over the age of two.

** Tully, K. P., & Ball, H. L. (2013). Trade-offs underlying maternal breast-feeding decisions: A conceptual model. *Maternal & Child Nutrition*, 9(1), 90–98.

*** Eglash, A., & Proctor, R. (2007). A Breastfeeding Mother with Chronic Breast Pain. *Breastfeeding Medicine*, 2(2), 99–104. TO READ.

****Buck, M. L., Amir, L. H., Cullinane, M., & Donath, S. M. (2013). Nipple Pain, Damage, and Vasospasm in the First 8 Weeks Postpartum. *Breastfeeding Medicine*, 9(2), 56–62.

us with another layer of understanding aversion: a mother's life with aversion and her desire to continue breastfeeding despite pain or discomfort, despite feeling trapped or 'touched out', despite the guilt and shame, is also actually simply biological.

Oxytocin (and stress)

Oxytocin is a rather marvellous hormone that is primarily known as a female attachment hormone as it plays such a large role in both birth and breastfeeding and is well known for being the key active ingredient in creating a lifelong bond, not only in mammalian sex behaviours, but also through mammalian milk feeding. Yet, there are less known mechanisms in the body that it affects. I certainly didn't know that the effects of oxytocin can make you incredibly thirsty, or can make you feel anxious. And anecdotally we know that addressing both hydration and anxiousness around breastfeeding can help lessen or even remove aversion. Oxytocin is also known to have this wonderful ability to reduce our sensitivity to pain and dumb down fear,[*] which can help us mothers carry the burden of maternal responsibilities of newborn care in the early days of our child's life. Kendall-Tackett and Moberg write that important hormones involved in lactation, like oxytocin, can help mothers tolerate breastfeeding.[**] It is known that many women enjoy breastfeeding and this is largely due to oxytocin. The idea is the more you let-down, the more oxytocin you feel, the calmer and more in love you feel. This may explain the honeymoon period at the newborn feeding stage for many women, and why aversion kicks in later on as the nursling grows, when milk production or volume is less, or the nursling suckles less frequently. But if your breastfeeding experience started stressfully or in pain, or you have experienced a traumatic birth, the same hormone oxytocin can actually trigger fear and even

---

[*]   Zak, P. J. (2013). *The moral molecule: The new science of what makes us good or evil.* London : Corgi.

[**]   Uvnäs-Moberg, K., & Kendall-Tackett, K. (2018). The Mystery of D-MER: What Can Hormonal Research Tell Us About Dysphoric Milk-Ejection Reflex? *Clinical Lactation, 9*(1), 23–29

pain, and may be the reason why you are experiencing aversion. Lesser known, but crucial in understanding aversion, is that oxytocin can also cause aggression by triggering the fight or flight response.[*] With such close special proximity, aggression and aggressive feelings are bound to have some overlap when breastfeeding. New research shows that oxytocin can be the cause of emotional pain too, because even though oxytocin has selective amnesic effects on human memory[**] (like forgetting childbirth), it is also the hormone that strengthens social memory in the brain.[***] This means if you had a stressful social event, or a stressful and negative experience, not only will the memory of these be strengthened by oxytocin, but you will have increased susceptibility to being fearful and anxious during stressful events in the future. And I figure that there are mothers who will have an array of stressful events ahead of them after having a baby – many related to breastfeeding itself. In the UK and US, with a culture of bottle-feeding and breastfeeding being frowned upon in many places in public, breastfeeding itself can be stressful, without mechanical or biological breastfeeding challenges! Perceived issues of milk supply can be stressful. Each growth spurt of a nursling can be stressful, particularly if you do not know about growth spurts and how intense and full-on they can be. Returning to work is stressful: figuring out how to pump, if you can't pump enough, how to store and give your milk, and whether or not to introduce formula. Then there is weaning from the breast. There is a reason why it is not recommended to introduce a bottle as your nursling gets to one year of age and over: the longer they use a bottle, the more they will become attached to it, and the harder it is to wean from. For many babies and children, attachment to a bottle can be similar to attachment to the breast. As your nursling gets older, any attempts to reduce or restrict breastfeeding can be very

[*]   Ibid.

[**]   Heinrichs, M., Meinlschmidt, G., Wippich, W., Ehlert, U., & Hellhammer, D. H. (2004). Selective amnesic effects of oxytocin on human memory. *Physiology & Behavior*, *83*(1), 31–38.

[***]   Guzmán, Y. F., Tronson, N. C., Jovasevic, V., Sato, K., Guedea, A. L., Mizukami, H., … Radulovic, J. (2013). Fear-enhancing effects of septal oxytocin receptors. *Nature Neuroscience*, *16*(9), 1185–1187.

stressful, particularly night feeds. It can all be experienced as stressful.

How we personally deal with stress, and how we outwardly respond to it, will play a role in whether we are enjoying breastfeeding and mothering, particularly if aversion strikes. And, of course, the stress pathway in our bodies is inextricably linked to the hormone oxytocin. In fact, the direct inhibitors of oxytocin are the 'stress' hormones, and given what we have just discussed about the two-facedness of oxytocin, it is not surprising that these pathways are in same part of the brain: the paraventricular nucleus. The paraventricular nucleus controls both pathways and the emotions that arise from them when they are triggered. Moberg and Kendall-Tackett write about this interplay in their paper about D-MER, stating that usually when one system is upregulated, like the relaxing effect of oxytocin when breastfeeding, the other is normally downregulated.[*] They posit that oxytocin can be paired up with a negative response in the breastfeeding relationship, and that this could account for the negative feelings experienced when a mother has D-MER. In light of this I wonder if this is what happens in women who get aversion: breastfeeding is triggering negative emotions because the oxytocin is negatively paired, and the stress system is being triggered. Lifetime experiences can dictate how you manage and deal with stress. The reason aversion arises in you is specific to you, because everyone is slightly different and has a different combination of personal preferences and personal thresholds. One key variable is your personal pain threshold, another is sleep deprivation, and a third is how sensitive you are to sensory stimulation.

Sensory sensitivity

We all have different levels of what makes us feel good, bad or uncomfortable. Auditory, sensory and visual sensitivities

---

[*] Uvnäs-Moberg, K., & Kendall-Tackett, K. (2018). The Mystery of D-MER: What Can Hormonal Research Tell Us About Dysphoric Milk-Ejection Reflex? *Clinical Lactation*, 9(1), 23–29. p24.

can mean that different women have different capacities to cope with what breastfeeding entails. Being affected by loud noises, strong smells and even bright colours can be hard for sensitive people, and highly sensitive people (HSP) who are emotionally sensitive, who get bothered when they have a lot to do in a short space of time and need to withdraw after a busy day to a quiet or darkened room.[*] Having these sensitivity traits can make mothering more difficult because, in effect, you are being persistently overstimulated by your nursling. By mothering and breastfeeding. Babies and children can be loud, often do not stop moving unless they are asleep, and have very different needs and preferences from their adult caregivers. Nurslings have different sleep cycles to their mothers, some babies cannot sleep without being on or touching their mother, and others sleep while being continually latched on all night. Some mothers cannot sleep while being touched or having their breast in the mouth of their nursling all night, but others can. An additional consideration for highly sensitive people is that they tend to be emotionally sensitive, and are good at social emotion absorbing. This is a positive quality, but in mothering can mean becoming easily overwhelmed by emotions; if they are perturbed by a crying nursling, they may even find it painful until the crying stops – until they breastfeed them. For HSPs, their pain is great pain, their joy is great joy and they cannot do things by halves, because it is not the way their minds and bodies work. Mothering is a rollercoaster for the senses, so aversion and its aftermath for these mothers is a like a mini hurricane of emotions. It is no wonder incessant suckling, stroking, pinching, or nipple twiddling can be tolerated by some, but for others, like HSPs, it makes them want to gauge their eyes out and causes rage. And this is similar for mothers who have misophonia – a condition characterised by a negative emotional or autonomic reaction to specific sounds – which is not uncommon in the aversion community.[**] Personal preferences and tolerances

---

[*]   Aron, E. N. (1999). *The Highly Sensitive Person: How to Thrive When the World Overwhelms You* (6TH PRINTING edition). London: Thorsons

[**] Palumbo, D. B., Alsalman, O., De Ridder, D., Song, J.-J., & Van-neste, S. (2018). Misophonia and Potential Underlying Mechanisms:

are undoubtedly a consideration when we try to understand aversion, its triggers, its causes and what can alleviate it.*

If you are emotionally sensitive as a person, it might be easy for you to put yourself in another person's shoes, and difficult for you to understand why others can't do the same. This becomes tricky when the other party is a baby or toddler. Although rationally it doesn't make sense, there is a kind of underlying hurt experienced when you don't want to breastfeed but your nursling does not accept it and does it anyway. Questions like 'Why can't you see I am in pain?', or 'Why can't you just accept that I don't want to be touched or have my breast in your mouth right now?' may go through your head. This inability of a nursling to empathise causes frustration and upset for a mother, as it would if an adult were to do the same: to be inconsiderate or rudely trample on your feelings. Coupled with having pain when breastfeeding, or overstimulation, it can mean the mother is in a state of persistent, often cumulative stress.

I know it makes no sense but what I needed was being ignored by her. She clearly didn't understand that my nipples felt like someone was using them on a cheese grater, even when I kept telling her it hurt. How could she? She was tiny. I had to be a silent martyr – no one could see the prison I was in. It was stressful, lonely and dark. Liliana, Russia

Mothers' accounts of aversion show that breastfeeding can and does trigger a stress response, not always because of the activity of breastfeeding per se, and not only because of previous life events and the role of oxytocin in replaying and intensifying them, but because of everything breastfeeding necessarily entails alongside these. It can be rather limiting and restricting to breastfeed, and this restriction or constriction causes festering frustrations to worsen. Anyone who has experienced being stuck breastfeeding to sleep during the

---

A Perspective. *Frontiers in Psychology*, 9. https://doi.org/10.3389/fpsyg.2018.00953
* We cover preventing and alleviating aversion in Chapter 8.

night knows that lying motionless in a dark room can bring our worst demons to the fore. And even though we know the benefits of breastmilk and the importance of breastfeeding, when we are in the thick of it we see no actual tangible reward. It's one thing to believe in sacrifice as a mother, another entirely to live with it. It is not like other 'work': we do not get a pay-cheque to offset the fact that we drag ourselves out of bed to get to a soul-destroying office job. We also have direct personal costs, as we often have no access to reasonable breaks and we have limited or non-existent personal boundaries. We also see no motivational benefits, as we have no pats on the back from colleagues and no spectators to marvel at our daily and nightly sacrifice. My analogies with work are not really analogies. I consider breastfeeding to be *actual work*, a job, that in the past would have earned you a lot of money if you became a wet-nurse. In the 18th century up to 80 percent of infants in Paris were sent to wet-nurses, often not in the same town,* and in Arabia wet-nurses were selected very carefully, highly respected and paid amply for their role. But who in their right mind nowadays would take a full-time job that causes you to be tired, grumpy, 'touched out', hungry and thirsty with no time alone, and not get paid for it? Mothers. Those who are just following what their biology dictates: post-birth, lactogenesis happens. Those with a sense of obligation and duty to their offspring who want to do the best for their child. Those who have been born into an age of an explosion of research into child development and child rearing, and those with an acute wariness about causing harm.

Finding good quality quiet time, when you experience no sensory sensation, can be very difficult, if not impossible, if you are a mother. Some newborns need to be held literally all the time, and everyone knows that toddlers will follow you to the bathroom or get into the shower with you while they are fully clothed just to do what you do, and be where you are. And this is normal for little people. Just difficult for mothers in the 21st century. Being a responsive parent can mean

---

* Drake, T.G.H. (1940). The Wet Nurse in France in the Eighteenth Century. *Bulletin of the History of Medicine, 8*(7), 934–948.

bed-sharing at night, after having constant contact, constant activity and noise during the day. There is no sanctuary that is yours, and no way to create lasting space, time, or a break. Add aversion into the mix and the fight or flight response can mean that emotions of fear, anxiety and sadness are rife: life can become rather unbearable for people that are sensitive to external stimuli, HSPs or on the sensory sensitivity spectrum, including those who are autistic.

Weaning

One of the most surprising things for me when I was breastfeeding was how hard weaning was. Or rather, was how unexplainably attached my children were to breastfeeding and my breasts. And this is true for many, many nurslings. And it's not the breast per se, as we know it can be to a bottle too. I have thought a lot about this attachment and how to explain it to mothers, because social theory states that negative feelings like anger can arise when there is a clash between expectation and reality. Understanding normal nursling behaviour can help redress that. Showing mothers what is normal when it comes to nursling behaviours and weaning can lessen or remove aversion. Expectations align with reality. To try to find terms and describe these behaviours, I borrowed from my academic and professional past.

I used to work for a public health department commissioning and managing substance misuse services. It seems to me that some of the behaviours of nurslings who are attached to breastfeeding are actually similar to those of an addict – the drug here being the milk. As with addiction, it is not just about the drug, or the dependence per se, but the ritual of getting it, the environment that you get it in, the triggers that make you want to use, the relief it offers you, and the whole attachment you have to the *process*. I find many parallels and similarities when thinking of breastfeeding for nurslings in these terms. Babies have an instinct to breastfeed, and this makes biological sense to survive, but there is a point at which it seems to become more of a habit than a need, and then the habit becomes a somewhat addictive kind of habit, leading to what can be described as 'addictive' behaviours. From being biologically normal for a newborn, later there can become an absolute dependence on breastfeeding to sleep, and the dose required also seems to increase for some nurslings, because even three hours of on-off breastfeeding to sleep doesn't work sometimes. These addictive behaviours, of sorts, can be seen in nurslings that are constantly searching for the breast, constantly asking for the breast, constantly attached (literally) to the breast, or never satiated after breastfeeding. Substance misusers use substances to get away from pain; they use substances to fill a void when they do not have a deep connection with themselves or others. Nurslings use breastfeeding when teething or in pain, and I wonder if the more intense behaviours in nurslings who demand the breast arise because they do not have a good connection at the time with their mother. Do they behave in this way because their mother is stressed, or 'doing other things', and her social nervous system is offline, resulting in the connection to the nursling being lost? Aversion itself can certainly cause a disconnect in the relationship, and affects a nursling's behaviour – as it can the mother's. Distracting yourself with your phone, or moving your attention elsewhere, means your social nervous system is offline: nurslings can become clingy and suckle more in response, which would certainly help keep the vicious cycle of aversion turning (as seen in Figure 3 on page 36).

Triggers are a common consideration in the description of addictive behaviours: there are also triggers to breastfeed for nurslings, and triggers for aversion for mothers. Breaking the 'habit' of breastfeeding could be considered tiresome and hard as breaking a habit of addiction, with repeated 'relapses' in your attempts to wean, as in the attempts to 'go clean'. Then, conceptually at least, there is the 'will' that is often written about in the literature of addiction. One famous philosopher conceptualised addiction as 'weakness of will', or the inability to remain resolute when needed. This will is a key factor in breastfeeding for the mother, to establish supply, and to continue to breastfeed, but also when it comes to weaning. The will of the child is also a factor, as for nurslings it is the 'will' to survive. The 'will' is a kind of resolve, commitment, or determination – and although we can't attribute a conscious *intention* to survive to young nurslings, reframing the tension and conflict that weaning can bring as a 'battle of the wills' helps us understand what is going on in a breastfeeding relationship dynamic, and why it is hard to stop breastfeeding. The will for a mother can be the commitment to carry on, or seeing through the decision to stop breastfeeding altogether. Both of these can be a difficult experience for a mother with aversion; although she may want to stop, she will be torn by emotions of loss and guilt at ending the breastfeeding relationship. For the nursling it's about the will to continue, and some have a very strong will and attachment to breastfeeding. When we think about weaning attempts, the one with the strongest will wins in the end in mothers with aversion. Now I am not saying nurslings are addicts, or mothers have weakness of will if they continue to 'give in' and breastfeed through aversion, despite wanting to stop breastfeeding. Just that conceptually, in an abstract form, as an idea, the language used in addiction theories can be helpful in plotting patterns and behaviours in a breastfeeding relationship that has started to experience tension. And framing it in a way that shows similar behaviours in other parts of the living world helps some mothers understand their nurslings.

Understanding these seemingly natural behaviours and connection to breastfeeding for nurslings can help bring the expectation of how nurslings 'ought' to behave back to reality. This is why it can help with aversion – because negative emotions can arise when your expectations do not match your reality. While some mothers can manage the process of weaning off the breast with more ease, perhaps because their nursling doesn't have a particularly strong will to continue to breastfeed, others categorically cannot, so this process does portray a negotiation aspect of the breastfeeding relationship, and the conflict that arises due to this. Parent-offspring theory suggests that children take more energy than parents are willing to or able to give, so conflict invariably arises. We see this often, even outside of the discussion of breastfeeding, in the behaviour of toddlers deemed to be challenging your authority, when it is a matter of who will 'back down'. While it may not be a pleasant way of understanding interactions between parents and their offspring, describing the daily interactions as conflicts is accurate for some families, with the tensions, tantrums and tears. And it is useful to think of these situations without ascribing judgement, moral value or blame, because it helps us frame how we understand our own interactions and behaviours. And, consequently, how to move past them and change behaviours that cause conflict to persist. Similarly, with nurslings who seem to behave in an almost *obsessive* way about the breast, and seem *addicted* to the milk, this characterisation is not meant to portray them in a negative light, but it gives us the words to describe their behaviours during that period. And if we keep it amoral – without ascribing any 'good' or 'bad' to their intent, and without holding them accountable for their behaviour – I think it is a useful way of framing why we can struggle with weaning. They are *dependent* on milk, on breastfeeding; and we are *depended on* to supply it. It is also useful when thinking about aversion as the biological start of weaning off the breast with older nurslings; this friction with the battle of the wills may need to occur in order for conflict to arise to reduce or restrict feeds.

When researching this book, I sought out papers about lactation and parenting in other mammals, because, as evolutionary biologist Katie Hinde says, 'mammals suck'. I wondered, as we are mammals, what other mammals did to wean their offspring off the breast? I read that sows will increasingly stop nursing as their litter gets older by changing their posture to hide their teat line.[*] I notice that humans end up doing this too: if push comes to shove, even in high summer we will wear completely covering tops to prevent access. I watched animal documentaries that showed a lioness batting her small cubs off her if she didn't want to nurse them, and a panda mother contorting and twisting her body, even getting

---

[*] Johnson, A.K., Morrow, J.L., Dailey, J.W., & McGlone, J.J. (2007). Preweaning mortality in loose-housed lactating sows: Behavioral and performance differences between sows who crush or do not crush piglets. *Applied Animal Behaviour Science, 105*(1–3), 59–74.

up and walking away from her baby, when she didn't want to feed. Of course, I cannot attribute thoughts and emotions to these animals, but it certainly looks like what happens when you get aversion. You stop, move away from, or have an urge to push your child off you. Yet the animal nurslings didn't seem to 'throw a tantrum', even though they are remarkably persistent in their requests for milk. And they are persistent, despite their mothers clearly indicating that they didn't want to or couldn't give it to them. In humans this is one of the main difficulties faced by mothers who have persistent aversion: the nursling tends to react badly to the mother's refusal to breastfeed. Repeated incidents of aversion or de-latching can mean that things escalate – without a consistent message of 'no', which the nursling would have if the mother weaned outright, the vicious cycle plays repeatedly. And without the 'village' around us as mothers, we do not know how to behave, or what to say or do to negotiate this conflict, and we may end up making the situation worse. For over 95 percent of our existence as humans we lived in hunter-gatherer societies, and we lived in consistently similar set-ups wherever we settled in the world. We had a sharing-based community, with well-established and maintained social constructs in which females would get help raising their offspring, both directly through milk-sharing, but also through other adults chiming in with parental responsibility, regardless of genetic relationships to children.* Hunter-gatherers practised alloparental care, or communal parenting, in which a child would know who its biological mother was, but any adult in the group would pick up a distressed or crying child. Imagine this in the context of a mother struggling with aversion and having to de-latch, or in the process of weaning: all those other adults to step in to give parental love and care. We would have a drastically different story to the one-on-one weaning battle we often see now.

According to Borries and colleagues, mothers and infants *negotiate* milk transfer. When the process of weaning begins, and how long it continues, varies across mother-infant pairs

---

* Ryan, C. (2011). *Sex at dawn: How we mate, why we stray, and what it means for modern relationships*. New York, NY: Harper.

or dyads.[*] I like the idea of weaning being a negotiation, because it can really help to discuss it with your nursling as if you were negotiating a deal – especially if you have aversion with an older child. Consciously having the conversation out loud, with your partner, with a friend, and with your nursling, even if they are a toddler, can help you weigh up the pros and cons of weaning, and makes the negotiating process easier over time. Small children are much more emotionally and cognitively intelligent than we as a society give them credit for. Weaning in an open, collaborative way can change the experience if nurslings are amenable, and if the mother has the energy and support to explore ending breastfeeding this way. As attachment-parenting *nurturing* mothers in the 21st century, weaning tends to take time, as it is difficult to see your nursling distressed and upset, and to know that you caused it by refusing the breast or changing breastfeeding habits. Ideally, many of these mothers hoped for self-weaning and aimed not to interrupt the process, but aversion kicking in changed this goal and they could not allow nursling-led weaning from the breast.

There are many biological reasons why weaning can happen, and we know that weaning is something that is more likely to happen as the age of the nursling increases. Wang and colleagues found that from the second year of life in children, there was a downregulation of the lactase gene, which is actually genetically programmed.[**] Lactase is the enzyme we have that breaks down lactose, which is the naturally occurring sugar in milk, so having less of it will mean it is more difficult to break down lactose. The authors posit that this could be a determining factor in why self-weaning starts, because the symptoms of lactose intolerance aren't exactly

[*]   Borries, C., Lu, A., Ossi Lupo, K., Larney, E., & Koenig, A. (2014). The meaning of weaning in wild Phayre's leaf monkeys: Last nipple contact, survival, and independence. *American Journal of Physical Anthropology*, *154*(2), 291–301 and Lee 1996.

[**] Wang, Y., Harvey, C. B., Hollox, E. J., Phillips, A. D., Poulter, M., Clay, P., Walker-Smith, J. A., & Swallow, D. M. (1998). The genetically programmed down-regulation of lactase in children. *Gastroenterology*, 114(6), 1230–1236. https://doi.org/10.1016/s0016-5085(98)70429-9

pleasant. Weaning can, of course, happen for other reasons: returning to work and the inability to express frequently, the introduction of a bottle or another caregiver, and biological favour by stopping tandem breastfeeding to prioritise a baby over an older nursling, to list a few.[*] Palmquist and her colleagues write about how an economic model can show how mothers will make decisions based on a trade-off of our interests and the baby's interest.[**] Deciding to wean is the result of weighing up the benefits of breastfeeding, with the cost it incurs from us as mothers. It seems we are not only political animals as Aristotle posited, but we are economic animals as well. With many mothers having demanding caregiving, work and family responsibilities, it is not surprising that mothers opt for paths that seem to need less energy and that are less time consuming: stopping breastfeeding altogether, expressing and using a bottle, or giving formula. Yet we do not know how much time it takes to breastfeed compared to formula feeding, and giving an approximate answer would be very inaccurate without looking at specific groups, as the time will vary for each mother-nursling pair. Sitting still for a breastfeeding session and not being able to move can be frustrating, but does it actually take less time to express milk, or make up formula, clean the equipment, store the milk safely and warm it appropriately in time for a feed? Maybe it doesn't matter, because the perceived freedom it gives may be enough to make a mother happy. We also don't know how much time it takes to wean an older nursling, as it can be time and energy consuming, and many mothers will delay weaning off the breast because it is simply too much effort. If a nursling is younger, many mothers feel that they are doing the child a disservice by weaning, and that they may harm their nursling by stopping breastfeeding. They may feel a lot of guilt even thinking about it, let alone going ahead with it.

Human breastmilk is amazing, full of currently uncreatable,

---

[*]   When to Wean | Mammals Suck... Milk! (n.d.). Retrieved 18 April 2018, from mammalssuck.blogspot.com/2015/01/when-to-wean.html

[**] Tomori, C.E.L., Palmquist, A., & Quinn, E.A. (Eds.). (2017). *Breastfeeding* (1 edition). Milton Park, Abingdon, Oxon ; New York, NY: Routledge. Chapter 14 & Chapter 11.

incredible and irreplaceable properties. This doesn't mean that breastfeeding for the longest time possible is *ipso facto* the best thing to do for some mother-nursling pairs. Dror Mandel and colleagues wrote that 'the optimal duration of breastfeeding is unknown'.* When I think of aversion, and the consequences of the physical, emotional and mental difficulties some breastfeeding mothers face when they have breastfeeding challenges, I wonder what the best thing to do is. The consequences of these challenges are unknown, as there is so little research: we don't actually know if is it better for these mothers to stop breastfeeding, all things considered. Sometimes I wish we did, so that the mothers who do want to wean but cannot justify it to themselves could have more accurate information with which to make an informed decision. We have a lot of information from research into the properties of breastmilk, the effect on maternal health, and the benefits for the child and even for society. We do not have very much research showing these benefits as weighed against the harms of not breastfeeding, or against the mother's specific experience. And even if we did, the process of weaning and its attributed challenges would need to be included in the trade-off decision-making. This would be tricky research to get right. Questions I would ask would include: how long will it take to wean? What impact does weaning off the breast have on the mother if she has to implement other strategies to calm and console her nursling, or to get them to sleep? Are mothers harmed by the emotional burden they experience when they continue to breastfeed through aversion? Are nurslings actually harmed if they are weaned off the breast before they are ready? Is it temporary or lasting harm? Perhaps there are too many variables to consider, and harm itself is not necessarily measurable, but because we know so much about the benefits of breastfeeding and the importance of species-specific milk, ideally from the nursling's own mother, the scales tip down heavy on the side of continuing breastfeeding for mothers, no matter what.

---

*   Mandel D, Lubetzky R, Dollberg S, Barak S, Mimouni FB. (2015) Fat and energy contents of expressed human breast milk in prolonged lactation. *Pediatrics*,116:e432–5.

But surely how a mother is feeling matters just as much as what a mother is doing? How you feel when breastfeeding must have some impact on your health, and dare I say even on your nursling's health? Even if we reframe the decision to wean off the breast as a choice between preserving your own health and providing the optimum food for your child, which may make the transition easier, acknowledging that it is an emotional and challenging change which can be just as intensive as establishing supply in the early days can make it a less appealing option. If only human nurslings could be like jackrabbit nurslings, who unusually for mammals only feed a couple of times a day from their mother and yet still thrive. Perhaps then we could be free of aversion.

* * *

I started this chapter by looking at some biological factors that could be causally contributing to aversion, and I will end it by looking at one last area: the consideration of what *kind* of women experience aversion, in our societies and modern life. The reason for this is because I consider aversion to be a biopsychosocial phenomenon. I want to know how much our modern-day lives, and the subsequent stress we experience, is affecting mothers with aversion and their nurslings. I'm also interested in how our lives before we became mothers relate to our lives as mothers. Take me, for example. I was a massive socialite as a young adult. I would often say yes to attending three parties or events in one evening, and then go on afterwards to dance the night away. It was probably easier because I didn't drink, so I would wake up feeling fine the next day and do it all over again, even after a full day's work. I always had plans: every night, next week, next month, next year. On weeknights I would be out; at weekends I would fly to Switzerland to spend time with my old university friends or go to stay at my childhood friends' houses around London or be back home in Norwich. At one point I was carrying on like this while working full-time and doing a Master's full-time! It started to become a bit unsustainable at that point, but I found it difficult to change my ways. I wrote my Master's thesis while travelling around Iran in the summer of 2005, which ruined both the travelling and the writing for me. I then started my PhD while working full-time and chairing a young person's charity in London. Around then things started to crack and my body started to give up on me, forcing me to slow down. As I did, I began to notice that it wasn't just me who was struggling with this fast pace. I don't know when life became the kind of extreme sport it seems to be now, but everywhere I look people are tired and running on empty, but still feel like they are not doing enough! Like many others I was caught up in the 'rat race': even without aspiring to more wealth and power, there is always something we *ought* to be doing, somewhere we *ought* to be, somebody we *have* to see, someone else we have to become.

In the 21st century it seems you aren't someone unless you are 'achieving' something or 'doing' something with your life. And with all the opportunity at your fingertips with online access to the world, it doesn't matter if you are a mother and mothering is a full-time job: there are really no excuses. This seems to be the underlying message, anyhow. It's overwhelming for many people, but as social mammals we tend to copy those around us, and seek their approval, even if it costs us our health. It also becomes addictive, as it is reinforced by social media: mostly people only post the extravagant or exciting parts of their lives, and the viral stories are of business successes and achievements against all odds. We copy, we emulate. A living human who is just 'being' is not enough anymore. Doing daily activities to sustain life or earn money is not enough anymore in society, so being a mother isn't enough anymore either. I'd go so far as to say that being a working mother isn't either, as there is always something more, something better, some other unattainable thing that creeps in. Mothers feel this pressure in the expectation to 'bounce back' to their old bodies, their old lives, and their careers. There is no time for mothering, and this means that there is no time for breastfeeding. It would be unwise to discount the affects this social pressure can have on us when we consider aversion.

This fast-paced life of self-pursuit and self-promotion in

the age of social media, in an era of individualism and *choice as king* is affecting everyone: us, our children and society. It leaves less time available for others – there is only a limited time in each day, after all. Perhaps because we each have a limited amount of energy, and mothering takes up rather a lot of it, we can no longer carry on 'achieving' as we used to. Then our self-worth unconsciously comes into question. This is reinforced by society and government policies that expect mothers to 'do more' and be someone else 'more important'. Returning to work and subsidised early childcare are national policies in the UK. There is a notion that you ought not be at home after your baby hits a few months old: the one thing a woman cannot do is be a mother, as it is not valuable or valued. Not only are we not rewarded or acknowledged as having an important role or doing an important job as mothers, but we also *feel* we are doing nothing. Yet this 'nothing', it seems, is a very hard thing to do. It is just a simple equation. Or, if you are a visual person, a breakdown of the slices of a pie chart. Everything you need to do in life (like eating, sleeping and work) takes a portion of the pie. Looking after the needs of another human being takes a hefty portion. Breastfeeding will too. Your time and energy is not limitless. I remember hearing J.K. Rowling say that in order to finish her first book some things had to slide, and the first thing to go was cleaning the house – for a whole year. Trying to do it all, and more, costs us. And that cost is experienced as stress.

The biology of stress

No longer are humans reliant on mothers to breastfeed their infants for humanity to survive, and no one knows this better than mothers. And if you were to think that this is a burden lifted, you would be utterly wrong. In fact, mothers now have both increased pressure to breastfeed and, at the same time, more options around infant feeding than ever before – which can make mothers worse off. The famous psychologist Barry Schwartz wrote about the 'paradox of choice', and although logic would assume that having more options is better for us, it actually increases stress and leads to poorer decision-making.* The onus is now on us to take responsibility for all our decisions, but we don't often have all the right information to make them, and we certainly do not have the right support networks to implement our decisions. To breastfeed, to wean, to return to work. Any and all of them, I would argue, can require a little additional help or they can become very stressful for some mothers.

Stress may have biological or evolutionary roots that are (at least temporarily) beneficial, but prolonged stress, and stress when you have no ability to change a difficult situation, is never a good thing.** Consider mothers who are juggling home life while battling a mental or physical health condition, or American mothers reluctantly forced to return to work at six weeks post-partum. Dr Gabor Maté said in a talk I heard: 'if women are stressed, their children are stressed'. Being stressed is often visible in our facial expressions and our body language, and we now know about emotions as social contagions that spread, through the social nervous system we all have as a way to respond to the environment around us and manage our stress. How does stress affect our breastfeeding relationship with our nurslings? Is aversion a manifestation of the stress a mother is dealing with inside? Does stress pass to our nurslings, or is there transference of it in our milk? How is stress affecting the dynamic and interaction between the mother and nursling? For me, the answers to all of these are key when considering the phenomenon of aversion. The milk is not just food.

Human survival is about more than just feeding babies: it is about attachment in the first years, and as a species at large it is about a kind of Hobbesian interaction and cooperation with others that we need and need to foster, in order to survive. Having aversion can and does jeopardise the process of attachment in arguably the most important neurocognitive developmental time of a human being's life: the formative years

---

*   Schwartz, B. (2004). *The paradox of choice: Why more is less* (1st ed.). New York: Ecco.

**   Payne, K.J. (2019). *Simplicity parenting: Using the power of less to raise happy, secure children*. Stroud: Hawthorn Press.

of early childhood. Breastfeeding is inextricably linked to the concepts of skinship and nurture, and how these foster love, connection and lifetime bonds that have been around since the dawn of human civilisation. When I first started to think about writing a book about aversion, in order to understand it better I realised I needed to understand how it all started. Had women always experienced aversion? Did cavewomen experience it, or tribal women? Did 1950s housewives struggle with aversion? I spoke to Penny Van Esterik, a professor of anthropology who has dedicated the last four decades of her life to researching infant feeding cultural practices, and author of *The Dance of Nurture.** She calls for us to move away from timed feeds and mechanical language when we talk about infant feeding: to dispense with volume consumed, weight gained, time spent. Then we can move back to understanding the nurture of our young conceptually as a dance: the giving and taking, the rhythm and movement, the love and the intimacy. Human civilisation has changed and evolved, and the way we birth and feed our offspring has too. We concluded that aversion likely had been around in history for many reasons, but that now it may be becoming more prevalent. Factors disrupting the natural biological processes of birth and breastfeeding, and preventing us from living as we used to in tribal and village settings, could cause a phenomenon like aversion to arise. In the 21st century, it seems, some women cannot dance the dance of nurture.

Historically, it is possible that some mothers may have experienced negative feelings when breastfeeding for some of the same reasons that mothers do now, such as menstruation, ovulation or persistent pain. Perhaps the experience of having negative emotions would have meant it was time to wean from the breast, or that another woman in the family or community took over breastfeeding the nursling, so not much thought would have been given to it. Milk-sharing used to be more common. Perhaps there were fewer expectations that

---

*   Van Esterik, P. (2017). *The dance of nurture: Negotiating infant feeding.* New York : Berghahn Books.

you would enjoy breastfeeding and be perfect at mothering, so when some mothers didn't enjoy it, they were not upset because their expectations didn't meet their reality. Perhaps these mothers weaned instead of breastfeeding through aversion, and didn't worry about the notion that it might harm their nursling's emotional or physical development, even if they cried for days. There was certainly less pressure to 'do' other things that weren't compatible with being at home and breastfeeding, and to 'be' someone else, some better version of yourself who is thinner, richer and happier. These observations led me to the next chapter in understanding aversion: modern life and how that affects our mothering, and motherhood in general. I cover how modern life affects our mood and our health, and how we understand ourselves in relation to society. And how all this plays out in relation to breastfeeding.

6

It's Just Society

I'm sitting on the bathroom floor, the shower is running, there is still blood from when I gave birth. When does this end? I'm so tired I would sell my soul for sleep. I haven't showered in days; he won't let me leave the room. He seems to just know, even in his sleep, he will wake as I sneak out to use the toilet. I'm only able to shower now because my partner is holding him. I don't want to go back to my room, and I am dreading the next feed. I am just praying he doesn't wake up after 20 minutes as usual, I can't bear the pain. I hate that he won't take a bottle. I'm so trapped, I hate breastfeeding. Why am I doing something when I whimper the whole entire time? Why does it all fall on me? Why is it so damn hard? Isn't it supposed to be easy? Anabella, Modena

If you are reading this book soon after first publication, you are breastfeeding – or interested in the subject – in an age when there has been an explosion of research in the field of lactation and breastfeeding. Along with recent findings in neuroscience and the revelation that our gut may be the master of the body, you will also have caught the last wave of the public health campaign 'breast is best' that served as a reaction to the last few decades of increased, population-level, formula feeding. With the rise of large companies that produce and aggressively market powdered milk, the change in working culture after the industrial revolution, and women entering the workplace, we have almost lost a whole generation of mothering knowledge on infant feeding. How many people did you see breastfeeding as you grew up? Did you help raise children and look after the family home as a young girl? How much time did you spend with mothers and babies as a young adult? What did you know about how babies behave and what they need before you gave birth to yours? For many of us the answers to these would be none, no, little and nothing. This begs the question, what *did* we think about mothering, motherhood and babies or children? Perhaps we didn't think much about these topics, but we certainly would have had ideas about what it was like. I wondered where we got those ideas from, and what they were. Why do so many mothers expect breastfeeding to be magical, or to be easy? I wondered how our ideas about motherhood, and how we expect babies, infants, toddlers and children to behave in a breastfeeding relationship, affect the breastfeeding experience. Rose writes about the utter silence on breastfeeding as a possible source of anxiety or pain, and notes that not every mother breastfeeds, whether it be out of choice, or because it is too painful, or because it does not work.[*] I wonder if this would be the case if mothers had more realistic expectations of breastfeeding, and mothering through breastfeeding?

Deluded Expectations

Years ago I took a class, and the teacher spoke about how ideas are formed: he told us about a *phantasm*, which is a mental representation of an object or thing. He spoke about having phantasms of growing up, thinking about what being an adult would be like, and how that affects our expectations of life. While I was doing some (seemingly endless) decluttering at home, I found my notes on this class and asked myself, what phantasms do the words 'mother' and 'breastfeeding' create in the minds of new mothers? What is the word 'breastfeeding' synonymous with in terms of our expectations? Recently I was

---

[*] Rose, J. (2018). *Mothers: An Essay on Love and Cruelty* (Main edition). London: Faber & Faber, p89.

very unwell for a few months, and I started binge-watching some of my favourite childhood programmes, one of which was *Friends*. The actors on *Friends* were the highest paid actors of all time; it was a very popular show. I don't know of a single person who, even if they hadn't watched *Friends*, didn't know about it. I began watching the episode where Rachel had her baby, and I realised that once she has given birth, you see the baby a handful of times and her life from then on is shown to be mostly unaffected. She does exactly the same things as she did before the baby, she looks exactly the same as she did before, she *is* the same. I had never noticed that before, and it made me pretty annoyed as I thought about it. Then I started thinking that this probably wasn't the first time that this had happened in a TV show, and I wondered how much images on TV or in advertising have affected what we think mothers do and what mothering is. How have we been affected, over time?

Modern students spend up to two decades – twenty years – in schooling and education without learning the basics of birthing and breastfeeding. Even with specialist education like medical school, most doctors often don't even know the simplest rule of supply and demand in breastmilk production and so make erroneous judgements and give incorrect medical advice to struggling breastfeeding mothers. Imagine if we knew more, imagine if our expectations matched the reality of birth and breastfeeding, imagine if we were prepared for it. I'm not saying it would wave a magic wand and make things easy. I am saying it could prevent the utter shock that you can experience when you become a mother, or the madness that you feel when you really have no idea what you are doing, and lessen the inability to cope or the feelings of depression that are becoming ever more prevalent. All these are appropriate responses to an impossible situation: going from being able to manage all areas of your life, to being able to manage none while also being responsible for the life of a tiny human being that you cannot walk away from.

'I didn't expect it to be this hard' is something I hear a lot when I ask about mothers' expectations of breastfeeding. And expectations play a big role in our happiness and in our ability to cope with life. Motherhood is no exception. What do we expect when we find out we are expecting? We might expect to give birth 'normally', we might expect breastfeeding to be 'natural' and come naturally to us, we might expect to fall instantly in love with our baby, and to be a great mother. We expect that our baby will stop breastfeeding so much when they start eating food at around six months, and then stop altogether of their own accord shortly thereafter. Perhaps we also expect that we can carry on being who were before we had a child, with bodily autonomy, agency over our actions and authority in our decisions. And these thoughts are coupled with images from magazines, adverts on TV and social media snaps. How many of these phantasms in our head are what we experience in reality? How many of these mental representations and expectations are crushed when we become mothers? I would bet that, one way or another, few mothers come out completely unscathed. The problem is that it is hardly ever possible to separate what we think about something from how we feel about it. That is where emotions and breastfeeding collide, and where I started to think about 'emotional milk': how our thoughts and emotions are inseparable.

Consider a common situation that many of us will have experienced. You have made plans to make a call or watch a film, maybe even go out, straight after your nursling falls asleep at bedtime. As the time for your plans edges closer, your nursling shows no signs of going to sleep, even though you have been in the room breastfeeding for nearly an hour. Your already mild stress levels rise further. Tension builds, your frustration peaks, your aversion is sky high, and everything spirals, meaning you have to cancel or rearrange. If it were any other night, and you had nothing in particular to do, and nowhere in particular to go, you would have been less stressed, less frustrated, and this would not have happened. It was in how you *expected* the scenario to play out that made breastfeeding to sleep more difficult that particular night. Expectations are not to be ignored when we consider aversion.

Your demographic status, and your socio-cultural

upbringing, can and does affect you and your expectations around motherhood, not only in how you think and why you think the way you do, but also in who you are and how you behave. Imagine you were born into a village in a pre-modern society, and you became a mother. Sure breastfeeding could be irritating or annoying at times, but would you have anger or rage, an urge to run away, or other symptoms of aversion? I am not so sure. Would you feel resentment about the life you lost, the person you were, and the fact you are being held back from being the person you could become? That's unlikely, because the individual pursuit of self and self-fulfilment is distinctly modern. Would you be frustrated by two-hour bedtime breastfeeding marathons? Or have anxiety every night about preparing for the next day's school run, and presenting your latest project at work to supervisors? These specific pressures in modern-day life simply did not exist back then, and exploring how they affect how we are as mothers and how we think as mothers is important in understanding aversion.

Modernity

Societal practices of parenting have shifted dramatically over the last few centuries. Few people are not a product of their environment, in the respect that the society we are born into determines how we understand and think about a topic. I used to think I was an independent thinker, had a strong will of my own and was little influenced by my environment, but after spending a few months in the Middle East after my degree, I found it much easier to wear a scarf and to own my Muslim identity over there. When I came back to the UK, after a few months I found I wrapped my headscarf differently: I felt less comfortable in it, almost as if I wanted to blend in with the norms of society, and my identity was slipping away. I have often wondered how I would have thought, and consequently felt, if I was born in a pre-modern time when birthing, breastfeeding, cooking and cleaning was all I was expected to do as a woman. You cannot say I would have been unhappy or discontented because I didn't have a career outside the home, because it might simply never have occurred to me. Imagine if you were born in another century, what would you do and how would you think? Very few of us would be thinking outside the expected societal norms and the status quo, as those that did suffered the consequences, and often made history books because of it, like Joan of Arc, Edith Cavell and Rosa Parks. I wonder whether a change in socio-cultural norms and normative behaviour from 'women at home' to 'women at work' meant we felt less of a responsibility to breastfeed and when we did breastfeed, we felt it was more of a burden.

Pre-modern women would have been expected to have sexual relations with their husbands when they initiated it, even if they didn't want to – it was part of marital conjugal rights. We now have sexual liberation, feminist thought and movements that have created expectations of mutual consent and enjoyment of sex. Having full sovereignty over your body, exercising total autonomy and giving explicit consent to be touched is now an expected norm. But with this expectation, and years of being able to exercise it, how does it feel when you become a mother and your bodily autonomy is necessarily compromised (by virtue of having a person that depends on you and your milk for their life)? We can't 'just say no' to our nurslings. Yet many of us have habitualised independence in our lives: it is ingrained in our decision-making and in our actions, and also reinforced by society. When you move into motherhood, this loss of independence and move into interdependence can be fraught with a deep personal struggle to break old habits. 'My breasts are my own' to 'my breasts are my nursling's' is a big shift, that even if our hearts and minds are willing to make, will no doubt require some unlearning. I am neither questioning the moral goodness of a pre-modern life or modern life, nor am I saying one is better than the other. I am asking, how did each of these eras affect us as mothers, how we understood mothering, and how we felt when breastfeeding?

The pre-modern person was bound by their duty and their place in the world. For many women, this would have meant being the home-keeper and taking the 'mother' role, basically doing all the 'home' work, including the birthing and raising of children. This was no mean feat, and a lifetime of work. Duty may have its own rewards even if you dislike it, but regardless of this, many women would have found peace in their role – even if it didn't give them meaning or financial reward. I say this not to suggest that life was better in a pre-modern world, or that it is worse now, but to suggest that it may not have occurred to many mothers that they could or should or would do anything different in their life. The life of a pre-modern woman was predetermined in many ways, and by being a mother she was doing what she was meant to be doing. The concept of 'doing otherwise' for self-fulfilment is a very modern development, and I would argue that it categorically affects our mothering ability, simply because it takes up time and energy. Doing more, being more, achieving more is part of *modernity,* which is a term used to describe the condition of social existence we find ourselves in now: an era in history that is characterised by scientific thought, and distinctly different to previous ages of religious or supernatural beliefs. Capitalism and wealth in modernity have brought about the age of individualism – a completely different age with different goals and pursuits.

Finding meaning in your life in a pre-modern context came from your upbringing, the place and family you were born into and the culture to which you became accustomed. It was not your choice; nor could you change it. If you were born to nobility, you were raised with class, had certain expectations placed on you, and lived a life of nobles – you couldn't choose *not* to be a noble. If you were born to parents who were rice farmers, you would become a rice farmer. Your father would have learnt how to farm rice from his father, and your mother would have learnt how to birth, raise children and help farm rice from her mother and the womenfolk around her. These roles would be the focus in the woman's life, and provide her with meaning, purpose and direction. Sharing responsibilities was common and many people in differing cultures in a pre-modern age lived in communities and worked together for protection and survival. This is perhaps another reason that milk-sharing and wet-nursing were more common in history, and are less common now with the move into modernity, capitalism and nuclear families. There are no 'tribes', no mummy 'villages' that operate this way anymore.

Modern life is almost the complete opposite of this past way of life, because modernity itself is *characterised* by individualism: the ability and right to choose what you do with your life. Finding meaning in modern life is essentially up to you, the individual. In this era of individualism, there is an expectation that you ought to pursue your own personal meaning and self-worth, and implicit in this is that *being a mother isn't enough*. It doesn't, no, it *shouldn't* define you. What is interesting to me is that the interplay between how we live as humans in each era isn't the moral or ethical judgement of which is better, but what has changed and what hasn't. One thing that hasn't changed from pre-modern times is that women birth, and of course that women breastfeed, and that women are overall still the primary caregivers. Yet what has changed is the fast-paced world around us: more is expected of mothers as individuals, and in turn, we expect more of ourselves. What this means is that mothers are stuck in a pre-modern experience with sole responsibility for motherhood, but in a modern world with modern expectations.

Our society told us choosing education and going to university was important, that careers were important, that living our fullest life was important. The same society makes mothers the object of too much attention or not enough attention when she needs it, either completely glorifying or overlooking maternal pain, and, as Rose writes, makes 'tormenting mothers its pastime'.[*] This society hasn't caught up to provide the structural support that would allow mothers to fulfil the fullest life we have been taught to aspire to since we were young. The same society banishes mothers from public places, and shames them for breastfeeding or bottle-feeding. The same society has governments that allow companies to

---

[*]   Rose, J. (2018). *Mothers: An Essay on Love and Cruelty* (Main edition). London: Faber & Faber, p3&9.

abuse the vulnerability of mothers by aggressive marketing of products that undermine mothering and put infants at risk.* Or, as Rose writes:

> *The radical care and visceral mess of child-rearing must neither degrade nor stain the upstanding citizen. The shameful debris of the human body, familiar to any mother, must not enter the domain of public life and spill over onto the streets.***

Mothers, it seems, must 'do it all', and 'have it all', like anyone in our modern and privileged lives full of opportunity – and a lifetime of education. Except they can't. For many mothers this illusionary vision is unattainable. And that fact is subconsciously, perhaps even consciously, crushing them.

Modernity gives people a sense of individualised self-sovereignty in almost all areas of their lives, but for women who are mothers I believe this creates a competing set of desires and feelings, a double consciousness, if you will. Double consciousness refers to a state where a person has problems with self-identification because they are unable to coexist the idea of two roles within themselves and do not wish to let go of either of them. And more often than not an attempt to integrate, results in loss of both. In modern life, it is important that you are free to choose, and that you feel free. These feelings entitle us to independence, which we can enforce with adults, but becomes harder when we consider our nurslings. Many women personally consider that their bodies are making milk for their nurslings, that the milk *belongs* to their nurslings, and aside from this mothers feel a strong desire to breastfeed, to respond to and to nurture their nurslings. Not only does this make aversion difficult to

---

*   The recalling of powdered formula milk as it contained contaminants that could kill babies, or the removing of sleeper products for sale due to infant deaths happens frequently. Quality control seems lacking in products sold to parents. See: Zurcher, A. (2019, April 13). Baby sleepers recalled in US after deaths. *BBC News*. Retrieved from https://www.bbc.com/news/world-us-canada-47917782.

**   Rose, J. (2018). *Mothers: An Essay on Love and Cruelty* (Main edition). London: Faber & Faber, p46.

deal with once it strikes, but this Catch-22 situation can mean that we are more likely to develop aversion. We feel at once biologically and emotionally compelled to do something that we are not socially acculturated to do, or don't feel societally comfortable with, which restricts us physically and demands a lot of our time (when we could be and indeed *should be*, doing something else). It is a manifestation of some sort of ongoing dissonance between what mothers' *bodies* are telling them – that lactogenesis follows birth and is a biologically ordered process – and what *society* is telling them – to be free, to be independent, to do what you want, whenever you want. Feminism is at its heart about the equality of men and women, and we want to advocate for it, but this society is one in which you have to earn money to be worthwhile, you have to be doing something else with yourself, not just being a mother, in order to be accepted as someone of value. There is still an overarching assumption in society's attitude that motherhood is easy – that it isn't 'work' – because only getting paid for something means it is worthy of your time and energy. Yet, having to work or return to work as a mother brings formidable challenges: aside from being separated from your nursling, there needs to be time to express milk or introduce formula, which brings its own difficulties. Feminism should really focus on equity rather than equality when it comes to mothers. The conflicting emotions that arise when you have to leave your nursling with another caregiver are very difficult for some mothers, as is coping with a day's work after little to no sleep the night before. It is biologically normal for babies and toddlers to wake at night, yet neither society nor the working world acknowledge this and accommodate it. And this is not even considering the time and energy it takes for personal somatic maintenance that we humans need (ie, 'me' time), to recover, regroup and recharge from the day's activities and requirements. Mothering itself is a combination of many jobs that are considered distinct in the modern world: cook, cleaner, nanny, teacher, nursery nurse – and mothers often do all of these with no respite and no proper breaks. In fact, breastfeeding itself, purely in terms of time spent, is nearly a full-time job. Breastfeeding for a year takes close to 1,800 hours

– if you were to work a full-time job with three weeks' holiday that would be 1,960 hours on average.* So in addition to already having a few full-time jobs, all of which many mothers have to do alone, in modern life you ought to get back to 'work' that pays you and that is outside of the home too. It seems a little absurd. Actually, it *is* absurd.

We know that tribal, indigenous and pre-industrial times saw shared burdens of parenting work with community food preparation, shared nursing responsibilities, and access to more than one trusted adult caregiver to respond to a child's needs.** With a little thought, it's common sense to arrive at the idea that motherhood *and* having a job places constraints on your time and energy that are much higher than those on a working individual who is not a mother. Not only does this mean that many mothers are constantly burnt-out, it also means that there is a constant level of stress in a mother's life. Because, if what I have detailed already isn't enough to make you stressed, then I can assure you that being responsible for a little human being that you cannot leave and you cannot just stop breastfeeding, day or night, is. And this is why so many women feel like they are held hostage, or feel like a prisoner when breastfeeding. They feel that they never get a break, and that they have no freedom, no rights as a person. They no longer have a sense of personal identity and are clamouring to get it back.

Loss of freedom in a society in which you are free

Freedom is in many ways linked to our identity, especially in modern life, because being yourself means being able to be free, so if you take away freedom you will essentially obliterate the person.*** When first becoming a mother this loss of freedom

---

*   Nelson, A. (2019a, June 19). *How to Make the Full-Time Job of Breast-feeding Compatible with Work*. Retrieved 8 September 2019, www.inc. com/amy-nelson/how-to-make-full-time-job-of-breastfeeding-com-patible-with-work.html

**   Grille, R. (2013). *Parenting for a Peaceful World* (Second Edition edition). New South Wales, Australia: Vox Cordis Press and the UNICEF Baby Friendly Conference lecture in 2015.

*** Gildan Media., Piero., & Ferrucci. (2018). *Your inner will finding per-*

can be a personal struggle for many women who have jumped out of the modern world, leaving their work or education, and are now drowning in the pre-modern world. Varying degrees of independence are lost, but feeling constrained is common, especially when exclusively breastfeeding. Having free will is a fundamental aspect of human existence, and to violate or restrict another's will is a legal crime, if not also a moral one.* Being able to choose what to do this very minute, as well as what you want to do with your life in general, is, in a modern world, fully acknowledged and celebrated. How does this aspect of free will play into our agency as mothers, when we have social duties and a duty of care to our nurslings? Although we can rationally understand that the obligation of breastfeeding nurslings is not actually impeding on our free will because we could just get up and leave, this does not take into account our feelings and emotions, nor those of our nurslings. Even though you may seem outwardly free to choose, as a mother the point is that you are no longer free of the consequences of your choice. So, for example, if you choose to stop breastfeeding at night, you have to find another way to get your nursling to sleep, or to stop them from screaming the house down and waking everyone else up. For many women who do not have help from a partner or trusted caregiver, these situations are both acutely stressful when they happen, and cumulatively stressful when they continue to happen – and they continue to happen because mothers either cannot or do not want to wean. Yet, at the same time they may need to temporarily or permanently stop breastfeeding as aversion has kicked in, and when severe the urge to de-latch and get away is very strong. This situation itself is very stressful, but I wanted to know whether this stress was happening in isolation in a mother's life and around her breastfeeding challenges with aversion, or if there were other external considerations. It seemed only natural to look at stress in modern life.

---

sonal strength in critical times. New York., p4.

*   Here I am not talking about 'free will' in terms of whether or not we truly have free will in a philosophical sense or whether all our actions are determined etc, but just the act of free will as experienced by us daily.

Stress as a 21st-century phenomenon

Stress that affects our health due to our lifestyle is a relatively new phenomenon, as the word was only coined by Hans Selye in 1936.[*] Although stress can be a good thing – a motivator to action, if you will – the Mental Health Foundation reports on a UK Government poll that found that around 74 percent of people have felt so stressed that they were overwhelmed or unable to cope.[**] The importance of our mental health and our ability to cope with life is becoming more apparent worldwide. There is an undeniable relationship between psychological factors and the experience of motherhood, and I would argue that this extends to breastfeeding too, because it is so much a part of motherhood for some mothers. In one study looking at breastfeeding and maternal support, 92 percent of mothers reported that they were mildly stressed,[***] so stress is a consideration when we want to understand aversion in our modern-day lives. Is the fact that breastfeeding takes time and energy, and that a lot of it takes place while sitting down and not moving, something that could trigger negative feelings? Absolutely! I ask instead, why *wouldn't* it? The world is moving faster than ever before. As a breastfeeding mother you are often literally sitting still, and metaphorically feeling as though the working and social world is leaving you behind. You are sitting still with a million things you *feel* you need to do that you cannot – and this is not just the irritating, unconscious undertone you perceive when the dirty dishes are piling up. For some women who have work commitments at home, or educational course deadlines, their ability to breastfeed and the time they can spend sitting down for breastfeeding sessions is reduced. If the nursling is not amenable or receptive and asks

---

[*]   Becker, B. A. (1987). The phenomenon of stress: Concepts and mechanisms associated with stress-induced responses of the neuroendocrine system. *Veterinary Research Communications*, 11(5), 443–456.

[**]   Mental health statistics: Stress. (2018, May 11). Retrieved 7 September 2019, from Mental Health Foundation website: www.mentalhealth.org.uk/statistics/mental-health-statistics-stress

[***] Jalal, M., Dolatian, M., Mahmoodi, Z., & Aliyari, R. (2017). The relationship between psychological factors and maternal social support to the breastfeeding process. *Electronic Physician*, 9(1), 3561–3569.

to be breastfed as usual, this can cause conflict and tension. I believe that these types of events and external stressors can trigger aversion, or make it worse in some women who have aversion for biological reasons.

Imagine you have a presentation to complete for tomorrow, you are on your period, and your nursling is taking three hours to settle for bed. You need those three hours to finish your work. What kind of response would you expect from a human under those circumstances? When you take on too much, either mentally or physically, the body will say no at some point.* Aversion, for some women, will be their body talking to them, telling them to stop breastfeeding. And although there is an argument for aversion as a natural trigger for weaning, for many women aversion will creep in and cause disruption if other pressures exist in their life. In some ways, this isn't so much a problem for the mother, but rather the other person at this party: the baby, infant, toddler or child. Their temperament and responsiveness to a change in the breastfeeding relationship dynamic dictates the breastfeeding relationship too, and they are affected by the messages and cues they get if the mother's negative emotions spill over, or she has to prematurely de-latch. Many nurslings depend on their mother to have a connection. They learn the world is safe from us, and if they get signals that show a break in that connection, by seeing their mother angry or stressed and taking them off the breast, they will want to be reassured and so ask to breastfeed again. Small humans need to go 'back to source', which is often the mother and her breast, and so it can become a vicious cycle. You may find that exactly this is happening: your nursling wants to breastfeed *more* when you are busy or stressed, and when you experience aversion. To understand why this happens we can look at how stress plays out, and how we humans respond not only to how the hormones flood our body, but also how we use the social nervous system to figure out what to do in times of stress. And

---

* Maté, Gabor. (2011). *When the body says no: Exploring the stress-disease connection.* Hoboken, N.J.: J. Wiley.

how mothers who are struggling, particularly at night, will not be able to do this.

Stress and the social nervous system

Stress can be contagious, and as breastfeeding mothers we are not exempt from stress and neither are our nurslings, because of *absorbed* stress. When trying to understand aversion in our modern society I believe it comes down to the interactions between three elements: the biological and psychological contributing factors, the socio-economic context, and the developed characteristics and preferences of the mother, even before she became a mother. Essentially, the likelihood of somebody experiencing aversion is not only down to their characteristics and social context, but for some women having certain life experiences too, not only currently but as a child. Questions I ask mothers to help them decipher the root cause of their aversion are things like: are you in persistent pain when breastfeeding? Have you been a victim of sexual abuse in the past? Are you struggling with day-to-day living as a mother in general? Is there a stressful life event happening, such as moving house, change in your job, or an educational course deadline? How is your relationship with your nursling aside from breastfeeding? Understanding the strength of the connection between mother and nursling can help unpick the cause of the aversion and help stop the vicious cycle continuing. Any lack of connection can lead to more frequent breastfeeding requests by the nursling and more time spent breastfeeding, so getting 'touched out' is more likely. And, as we have seen, this can trigger a stress response. But it isn't as simple as 'fight or flight', or the effects of a negative association with oxytocin. The fight or flight response is more complex, because we have a social nervous system which is controlled by a series of cranial nerves, which respond to and are affected by our environment, our connections to other people, and even the way we perceive these things. This *polyvagal* theory is based on the fact that our behaviours, and our health, have been shown to be impacted by our social circumstances.[*]

---

[*]   Porges, S. W. (2001). The polyvagal theory: Phylogenetic substrates of a

In order to understand this theory, we look at how nerves are engaged whenever we are in a particular situation. When the fight or flight response is triggered, you may not know that we look to others to understand and decide what we should do in a situation of perceived threat. Before we either engage the threat or run away, we will read the level of risk by looking at other people's responses for safety cues to see if the threat is real or not. Basically, the level of stress we feel is affected by how others are behaving and how others are dealing with the same situation. We may experience this when we ask other breastfeeding mothers about what is 'normal' or if we are 'doing it right'. If we get responses that are similar to what we are going through we begin to calm down, we feel a sense of relief, a feeling of belonging, and our stress about a particular issue reduces. I have witnessed this often in breastfeeding support groups: I can visibly see mothers' shoulders relax when they are told they are doing it right. Or when they come to the group struggling and say that the baby is always crying at home and doesn't latch, but we can get them to latch and breastfeed beautifully while at the group. I have often wondered whether this is down to expert support, or because both the mother and the nursling are less stressed at the groups. Others are around to reassure, smile, and make cups of tea or offer an ear. The social environment there is conducive to a mother to breastfeed. And interestingly, the series of cranial nerves that are involved in the social nervous system are the same ones that are integral to breastfeeding: the nerves linking the face to the tongue, and the jaw. These lead to the suckling reflex, swallowing, the digestive system and finally the gut. Stress affecting the social nervous system in a mother will directly affect her and her nursling's breastfeeding ability and experience. So what happens to this nervous system when aversion strikes?

To illustrate what may occur we can take an example: a mother who is a survivor of abuse may feel a perceived threat because she is frequently triggered. When breastfeeding at

social nervous system. *International Journal of Psychophysiology*, *42*(2), 123–146.

night, in a dark room, her nursling may clamber towards her breasts. She may have heard a noise and been woken abruptly from sleep, and before she understands what is happening her accessory nerve will make her turn to look around – a bit like when a deer freezes and looks to see if there is a predator nearby. Then there is a feeling of a sudden rush, it could be a mini wave of panic for a moment, and it is at this point that her facial expression will change. She may be scanning the room unconsciously for another person to check she is okay, or for another option to see if she can see a way out. A split second is all it takes for all of this to happen and for her to weigh up the situation, realising she is stuck with no other choices. While her body is realising it may need to flee, the vagus nerve removes the vagus brake from her heart and her heart rate increases to mobilise her body to get away from the threat. Her anxiety will increase internally, and her facial and bodily muscles will mirror this emotional state. This is a textbook stress response to a perceived threat, which I have applied to a breastfeeding mother who is alone at night, and is triggered.

Nocturnal adrenalin is then running through her veins. It is what our primitive, reptilian response would be in a cavewoman-type stress situation, in which, typically, the social nervous system would work to counteract this and neutralise any perceived threat. Seeing another person's face that seems calm or relaxed, hearing a calm voice or being told with a smile 'Don't worry, it's normal. I am here with you', changes everything. A calm touch, or someone you can see who is there to step in, offering the mother options of support and reassurance, will mean the vagal brake is reapplied. In this scenario a mother's heart rate would decrease and biological homeostasis would slowly return to her body. Her mind would reassure her that the situation is safe: the social nervous system would have been activated.

This theory was developed by a psychiatrist named Stephan Porges, who is known for proposing the concept of *neuroception,* which is our subtle detection of risk. From this theory, others hold that the nervous system controls our behaviours.* This brief outline of the theory can help us to understand why stress in modernity may affect us, because everyone has something to do, somewhere to be, and work to be done. Seeing people rushing around, late and anxious, may mean our stress response is always on, albeit at a low level. Porges also wrote about the face-heart connection: when our social nervous system is engaged, we talk, smile, and interact with cooperation. Our responses mirror our state: if we are safe and happy our feelings are of being calm, relaxed and in a loving safe environment. We can see this play out when our nurslings want to breastfeed and, how, when this connection is *not* engaged through the social nervous system, we respond to a situation very differently. For example, when you are trying to make a phone call to get that paperwork sorted or you have to make an online payment by a deadline, but your nursling is pulling at your top trying to get milk. At that time, you are trying to focus on something else, and you are not socially attached to and engaging your nursling. This means that your social nervous system will be slightly off cue, your breathing will not be as relaxed as your heart rate is a little elevated. Another thing that happens is that your middle ear muscles are not listening accurately to the pitch of speech (or pre-verbal cues) of your child's requests. Your nursling's interruption will be perceived or processed by your mind as an obstacle, you will become irritated, and you will respond in an irritated manner. This kind of response can in turn make your nursling more unsettled and persistent in their requests, because they too have a social nervous system that relies heavily on us as they look for cues and safety signals. They will pick up on your subtle stress signs and be affected: if you cry, they cry, you shout and scream, they will shout and scream. If you have a paroxysm of rage, so may they. Perhaps not at the same time, but they will certainly mirror your behaviour. Low-level stress in mother and nursling will seep out through language, body language, pitch or tone, and facial expression.

If we consider the beginning of the story for a mother –

---

* Fortuyn, J. D. (1979). On the neurology of perception. *Clinical Neurology and Neurosurgery*, *81*(2), 97–107.

pregnancy and birth – we can identify many factors that can interrupt the social nervous system. Women who are stressed or anxious during pregnancy tend to be stressed after giving birth, and one in six mothers develop anxiety.* Trauma and stress in pregnancy could possibly affect breastfeeding by changing the effect oxytocin has. In an animal study Hillerer and colleagues found that stress in pregnancy can actually reverse the positive effects of oxytocin when suckling** and can trigger a defensive, negative response – exactly what we see in the phenomenon of aversion. Birth interventions, and the drugs used, can also affect the mother-baby relationship. Synthetic oxytocin, which is often routinely used, is linked with an increase in postnatal anxiety and other mental health disorders.*** After birth, women are faced with a mass of information that is in direct contradiction to biological norms, breastfeeding norms and normal infant development and behaviour. These include being told to supplement with formula without being told it could affect supply, or to separate nurslings into their own room at night in order to force them to sleep and to ignore the requests of older nurslings because breastfeeding will harm them or has no nutritional benefit. If you start to research these kinds of comments, or even advice given by healthcare professionals, you begin to find an array of what seems like evidence to support contradictory claims. We live in an age in which we are free to do what we want, and free to choose how we parent, but we are then bombarded with information that makes it impossible to do that without having doubts and subsequently experiencing stress about those

* Ali, E. (2018). Women's experiences with postpartum anxiety disorders: A narrative literature review. *International Journal of Women's Health*, *10*, 237–249.

** Hillerer, K. M., Reber, S. O., Neumann, I. D., & Slattery, D. A. (2011). Exposure to chronic pregnancy stress reverses peripartum-associated adaptations: Implications for postpartum anxiety and mood disorders. *Endocrinology*, *152*(10), 3930–3940.

*** Kroll-Desrosiers, A. R., Nephew, B. C., Babb, J. A., Guilarte-Walker, Y., Moore Simas, T. A., & Deligiannidis, K. M. (2017). Association of peripartum synthetic oxytocin administration and depressive and anxiety disorders within the first postpartum year. *Depression and Anxiety*, *34*(2), 137–146.

decisions. Stress comes in many forms, and it is important to identify them.

Living without extended families, in a nuclear way, adds to the stress of parenting. Mothers are often alone and isolated with a newborn, perhaps with a toddler or other older children at the same time, and trying to meet the needs of all of them. At the same time they are not able to meet their own basic needs for adequate sleep and nutrition. It is naive to think that these pressures and stress do not affect the breastfeeding relationship. Stress itself manifests in bodies, notably in disturbed sleep and reduced sleep quality. And it is not just biological, but physical changes in our bodies too: stress can cause us to tense our shoulders, and this in turn affects positioning and attachment of a suckling nursling. Stress also affects infant behaviour and temperament due to the social nervous system. Some babies feed better at night or in a dark room than in public, or in the day when the mother is busy – why? It could be that they are easily distracted, but for those nurslings that aren't, it could be because it is a less stressful environment and the mother's biological and social nervous system is responding to this. Toddlers who are receiving stressed cues may start to feel unsafe, and will naturally go back to their safe space, the only constant they have known – the breast. Yet, for a mother who is stressed, this situation can mean that aversion gets worse, as a toddler can become more demanding when aversion strikes; when you are 'touched out' and unable to 'give more'.

The impact of stress is a big consideration when thinking about the capacity and ability of a mother to breastfeed. If breastfeeding were an actual contracted job, you would be remunerated and supported to do your job. You would have a manager, a clearly defined role, support and infrastructure, access to human resources, work safety assessments, and respite breaks as a basic human right. Yet many mothers have none of this, neither in kind, nor literally. And while 'their smiles are enough' to make it worth it for some mothers, it simply is not the case for other mothers who are struggling to the point of desperation and despair. It is little wonder aversion sets in for these mothers. It is little wonder anger and agitation manifest when these mothers have to sit and do an activity that prevents them from doing other (often necessary) chores or work, that prevents them from sleeping, eating, or even going to the toilet. Can these mothers do these things, are they physically able to? Sometimes yes of course they can, but what we need to consider too are the *costs* of doing them, and how these costs affect the whole family. A crying baby? A chronically overtired toddler? Weaning from the breast earlier than wanted? If we consider the role of breastfeeding in nurture and skinship we have the possibility of compromising these too. If we consider breastfeeding as a tool, we have the reduction of its use if you 'just say no', or prematurely de-latch and go off to do what you need to. This is problematic, especially if we consider the tool of feeding to sleep. The hours of time and all that energy spent getting your infant to sleep will be lost, the repercussions of an overtired toddler will wreak havoc on the rest of the day, and certainly the rest of the night with more frequent wakes. A breastfeeding mother who 'decides' not to breastfeed may suffer and struggle while she tries to manage her nursling's behaviour and wellbeing, and then her mental health will slide as there will be no wind-down time for herself. Winding down that can come in the form of quiet time when sitting and breastfeeding! Thus, mothers often make a quick assessment: they will forego eating proper food and responding to their body's toilet needs, they will forego sleep, and they will do what has to be done without much choice in the matter, because if they don't, they will pay for it in another way. Decisions mothers make that feel like a zero sum equation – a situation in which one person's gain is equivalent to another's loss, so the net change in wealth or benefit is zero – will always entail some amount of stress for one party. Here, it is the mother. The nursling is the one that gains, as all the mother's efforts are directed at meeting their needs. And even when mothers try to do this to optimise the home environment, they don't always win. They may have forgone everything to make sure their nursling naps and then the postman will knock so loudly that the nursling wakes up anyway, despite all their efforts. Then no one benefits from the mother's personal sacrifices, which can be frustrating and stressful too. The daily juggling act of trying to balance her own basic needs with the needs of her nursling(s), other children and other responsibilities can be extremely stressful for some women. And it isn't only the stress itself, it is how mothers personally manage stress, and if their minds and bodies respond negatively that is key when we think of aversion.

Stress can come from so many sources, often at the same time. We are not only interested in only those for breastfeeding mothers: I think it is important to know about stress sources from *before* women were mothers, and their ability to cope with stressful situations throughout their life. With constraints and loneliness, both of which mothers face, humans come face to face with no one but themselves, and in challenging times, like breastfeeding through motherhood, it is easy to be triggered by past events. You may feel particularly sorry for yourself at night as rumination is common at this time. You may find yourself recalling a traumatic event as a child, a death in the family when you were growing up, a painful breakup, or the loss of a job. Or you may be reliving a traumatic birth. Such events can have long-lasting impacts on mother-nursling relationships, and often mean women struggle more with motherhood. Birth can be a harrowing experience that many women retell as a kind of horror story for the rest of their lives. And if this wasn't bad enough, medical interventions are often done carried out without fully informed consent from women, perhaps because the side effects were not disclosed or discussed. For example, mothers who have the synthetic version of oxytocin to augment their labour find it more painful and have significantly more postnatal depression and anxiety compared to mothers that don't.[*] In addition, mothers who have synthetic oxytocin during labour are more likely to have epidurals, which block the release of naturally occurring oxytocin during birth, and therefore increase the risk of

---

[*] Kroll-Desrosiers, A. R., Nephew, B. C., Babb, J. A., Guilarte-Walker, Y., Moore Simas, T. A., & Deligiannidis, K. M. (2017). Association of peripartum synthetic oxytocin administration and depressive and anxiety disorders within the first postpartum year. *Depression and Anxiety*, 34(2), 137–146.

depression after birth.*

Sometimes, determining the exact origin of stress or trauma that is triggered is not as important as recognising that a natural system has been disrupted, and understanding what steps need to be taken to counter the disruption. As you become a new mother, sometimes you do not know why you are struggling, but research into the impact of birth interventions and the effects of our society means the reasons are becoming clear: we are interfering with the biological norms of birth and breastfeeding, with ripple effects across the mothering journey. One of these ripples, I believe, is aversion, because even though a certain amount of stress is normal and even useful at beginning of motherhood, so that we ensure our offspring survive, it was not as prevalent in mothers' everyday lives as it is now. Nor were women left alone to deal with it. Many cultures have the practice of 'rooming in' with a newborn for up to six weeks, with womenfolk tending to the mother's needs and duties so that she can focus on her nursling. This practice is slowly fading as other priorities of modernity take over for families, even in very traditional cultures like my own in Iran.

An increased, ongoing level of stress at the start of mother-nursling relationship means that the relationship takes a different trajectory – one on which the mother is more at risk of having anxiety and depression and, I believe, more likely to experience aversion. Some argue that it is helpful to divide the common sources of stress into two categories. The first is mental stress, which is characterised by worries and fears – like worrying about friends, family or work. The second is physical stress – from a poor diet, poor sleep or overexertion. Others argue that *both* these forms of stress can ultimately lead to fatigue, irritability and negative emotions, and make you more vulnerable to suffering poor health. This is because the mind and body are so closely linked that any symptoms of physical ill health can arguably be traced back to your mental

---

*   Kendall-Tackett, K., Cong, Z., & Hale, T. W. (2015). Birth interventions related to lower rates of exclusive breastfeeding and increased risk of postpartum depression in a large sample. *Clinical Lactation*, 6(3), 87–97.

health, and vice versa. In many ways they are completely inseparable. We know stress affects pregnant women, and mothers, so why not breastfeeding? As we covered earlier, Moberg and Kendall-Tackett write about the little-known condition of D-MER and state that depression, anxiety and negative feelings are increased with an upregulated stress response.[*] With aversion, I wonder if there is an over-stimulated stress response happening too, with hormonal pathways like those of oxytocin reinforcing the response. The relentlessness of mothering in the 21st century, with mothers' personal triggers including external factors and psychological factors stemming from childhood, may lead to breastfeeding itself being *experienced* as stressful when it is designed, at least biologically, to be the opposite.

Both our primal stress response triggers in the fight or flight response, and the cumulative stress of modern life, are factors to consider here. Although the immediacy of threats and dangerous environments arguably no longer exists in modern-day life, the biological pathway is still activated all the time. What happens when it becomes ingrained? When being reactive to a perceived threat becomes entrenched in our behaviour, in our body and cell memories, as a mother? If you are a mother who experiences aversion repeatedly, and it triggers a stress response, how does this affect you overall? There is an argument that mental and physical attrition when mothering, and the cumulative costs mothers bear over time, can negatively affect them.[**][***] This leads me to a large body of research and a growing movement that has yet to fully integrate into mainstream medicine, which claims that disorders and health conditions are all attributable in one way or another to a combination of three factors: biology, psychology and sociology.

---

[*] Uvnäs-Moberg, K., & Kendall-Tackett, K. (2018). The Mystery of D-MER: What Can Hormonal Research Tell Us About Dysphoric Milk-Ejection Reflex? *Clinical Lactation*, 9(1), 23–29.

[**] Spence, N. J. (2008). The Long-Term Consequences of Childbearing: Physical and Psychological Well-Being of Mothers in Later Life. *Research on Aging*, 30(6), 722–751.

[***] Luthar, S. S. (2015). Mothering mothers. *Research in Human Development*, 12(3–4), 295–303.

Biopsychosocial phenomena

Health problems and diseases are not isolated phenomena of individual human beings, they are also part of a society's culture; they are culturally manufactured. The biopsychosocial model of understanding health conditions involves considering a combination of social and psychological factors and how they are interconnected with our biology as humans.[*] We looked earlier at modernity, how it promotes individualism and 'achievement', and how this invariably leads to the persistent experience of varying levels of stress. Whether it's from having to work or study in order to afford to live, or being accepted by society, or watching others have to do this, the stress is always there.

We live with an artificial construct of time in our working day that ignores the seasons of the year, the patterns of the female body and the changes in a human body over time. Especially as mothers, with newborn rhythms, and often older children, we were not designed to be squeezed into rigid time structures and this causes us to have a deep mistrust in our bodies and our ability to mother.[**] A society that cuts us off from ourselves in a normal human state cuts us off from connection, not only to ourselves but to others, because it ignores our emotional needs. A society that idolises individualism and working can destroy social contexts – we see this ever more clearly in the rhetorical question mothers often ask: 'Where is my village?' Yet, this is just the nature of an economic system that doesn't value who you are, but what you can produce and consume, and how you are valued by others in society. People who do neither, in our case mothers, are devalued or even ostracised.

Many authors have written about how there is a rejection of women when they become mothers and are no longer in the workforce: mothers have to 'hide' their motherhood and their children from the working and public sphere. A public display of breastfeeding, although legal and apparently encouraged,

---

[*]   Lehman, B. J., David, D. M., & Gruber, J. A. (2017). Rethinking the biopsychosocial model of health: Understanding health as a dynamic system. *Social and Personality Psychology Compass*, 11(8), e12328.

[**] Dykes, F. (2005). 'Supply' and 'demand': Breastfeeding as labour. *Social Science & Medicine (1982)*, 60(10), 2283–2293.

is often frowned upon. There are specific places where children are acceptable, but the mother who attempts to go elsewhere and interrupts the value-adding people of the world is often punished. I remember the shame and then outrage that I felt when my friend and I were asked by a customer to leave Starbucks as our toddlers were running up and down disturbing those who were working in the cafe. I felt upset and angry that the lady felt she even had the right to ask me to leave: it was not her establishment, and it was certainly not only for working people. And this is not uncommon. People in society do not want to see or hear babies or children where they work, study, or relax, and many don't want to see mothers breastfeeding at all. It is not difficult to see how this generates a separation from ourselves as mothers, a dissonance in our character, a splinter in us that we can't quite find, but that continually irritates us. Where we once strived to become accepted and a part of society by educating ourselves and entering the workforce, consuming and having a social life, we now find ourselves to be utterly excluded, then isolated after giving birth. It can be a quiet life of desperation that we thought women had left behind. Loneliness prevails.

With nearly nine million people in the UK saying they are lonely, the ever-increasing loneliness in our society is recognised as having wider effects on individual mental health and the community as a whole.[*] Loneliness that mothers feel, day or night, when they have no one to talk to and no one to help, can create a deep psychological wound. Slowly realising that your life will never go back to how it was is a long, difficult and sad realisation that deserves time and a safe space to process. For a mother, this space is difficult to create for herself, with the burden of care and the responsibility for nurture. Mothers who struggle can feel ever more restricted and disconnected from their role when there are unresolved personal issues. And set against the idealised picture-perfect notion and images of motherhood we have grown up with,

---

[*]   Action on loneliness. (n.d.). Retrieved 7 September 2019, from British Red Cross website: www.redcross.org.uk/about-us/what-we-do/action-on-loneliness British Red Cross and Co-Op Published Report, 2016

we experience a daily sense of failure. However, we are often not aware of how our mind reacts to failure. Most of us have a default set of feelings and beliefs that are triggered whenever we encounter setbacks and frustrations. Our mind will try to convince us that we are incapable of something and we believe it. We will then feel helpless and we will stop trying too soon, or end up not trying to change things at all. Thus, we will become even more convinced that we cannot succeed, because as humans, if we become convinced of something, it is very difficult to change our mind. And it is just as hard to stop rumination – the cycle of negativity and the repetition of negative emotions and thoughts – which is common when we look at the vicious cycle of aversion. The shame and the guilt that follows aversion, the feeling of failing as a breastfeeding mother, hurts more and takes longer to recover from. Without connection to others, in a deep and meaningful way, we cannot easily break out of these cycles. Some women do not even know it is happening. And this is the case for many postnatal conditions like depression and mood disorders.

Pseudo-connection may exist in the form of social media, and this leaves you with a mini dopamine hit, one of Facebook's well-known integral designs that keeps you coming back for more, along with the endless scroll of the news feed. In short, it is addictive. And without any other tangible connection for many new mothers, it's sometimes their only connection with the outside world, but a rather warped one:

> *Being a mum has meant my friends have dropped out of my life one by one, and I am so alone. Everyone looks like they are loving being a mum online, but I really hate it. I think it makes me resentful when I'm breastfeeding. I am stuck at home because of it.* Liliana, Geneva

Not only on a macro societal level, but also in our microcosms in the home, this disconnect has had widespread effects. Screens, full-time working parents, individual rooms and even central heating are blamed for the poor development of infants and children – all of whom will be the adults of the next generation.[*][**]

Modern societies will generate pathologies because they do not allow your body to develop as it should, nor do they allow you to create an optimal response to situations you find yourself in. As a mother, when you are alone and struggling you can spiral lower pretty quickly without someone else there, and without your social nervous system online. Your assessment of a situation may become skewed, your anxiety rises, and you become full of stress, affecting your response to daily situations. Despite new-found freedoms in modernity, particularly for women, birth, breastfeeding and motherhood still present formidable challenges. Women are still at risk when birthing, they are still at risk in the postnatal period and mothers are not often considered as a vulnerable group in nationwide policy. The phenomenon of aversion is testament to this: the manifestation of negative feelings, being agitated and angry when breastfeeding, and having the urge to remove a suckling nursling all point to a kind of self-preservation. Breastfeeding mothers who are struggling in modernity are trying to exercise their autonomy when they feel trapped – for their own sanity – because the transition to parenthood is considered one of the most demanding and stressful life changes we face.[***] And depending on how you are able to manage and deal with stress, it is not surprising that when making this transition, a sense of control will predict symptoms of anxiety and depression.[****]

---

[*] Allen, L., Kelly, B. B., Success, C. on the S. of C. B. to A. 8: D. and B. the F. for, Board on Children, Y., Medicine, I. of, & Council, N. R. (2015). *Child Development and Early Learning.*

[**] Mustafaoğlu, R., Zirek, E., Yasacı, Z., & Razak Özdinçler, A. (2018). The negative effects of digital technology usage on children's development and health. Addicta: The Turkish Journal on Addictions. *(5) The Negative Effects of Digital Technology Usage on Children's Development and Health.* www.researchgate.net/publication/325263798 [accessed Sep 07 2019].

[***] Cowan, C.P., & Cowan, P.A. (2000). *When partners become parents: The big life change for couples.* Mahwah, NJ, US: Lawrence Erlbaum Associates Publishers.

[****] Keeton, C.P., Perry-Jenkins, M., & Sayer, A.G. (2008). Sense of Control Predicts Depressive and Anxious Symptoms Across the Transition to Parenthood. *Journal of Family Psychology : JFP : Journal of the Division of Family Psychology of the American Psychological Association (Division 43), 22*(2), 212–221.

Part IV

Urges of Autonomy and Survival

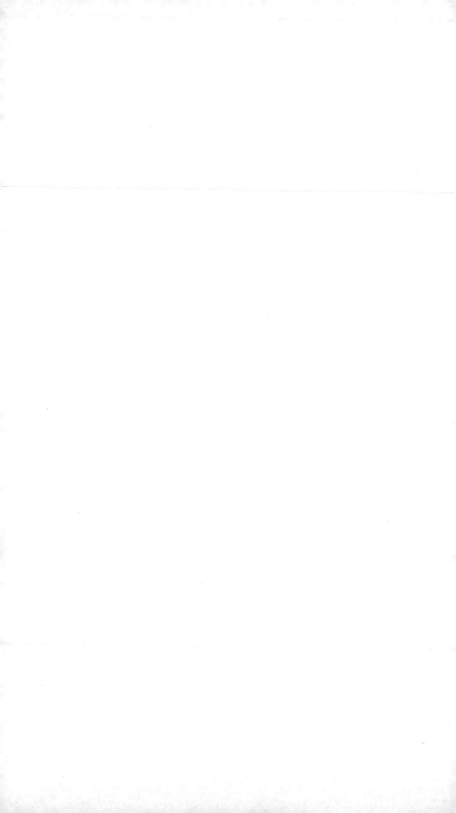

7

It's Just Psychology

We know how to maintain our physical health, and to take immediate action when we injure ourselves, but many of us know little about our psychological health and how to maintain our emotional hygiene. Psychological injuries, just like physical ones, can become worse over time if we ignore them. For a survivor of previous sexual abuse who is triggered by breastfeeding, with aversion becoming worse and disrupting the family home, this psychological injury can have an impact on her day-to-day life years after the trauma has happened. Sometimes, half the battle is recognising that the emotional and psychological injuries are even there to begin with, while the other half is to get through them without life-threatening wounds, to survive in one piece.

For some mothers who experience aversion I believe it is the manifestation of the urge of autonomy. Autonomy is the ability to choose to act without coercion or duress. It is a much-discussed concept in literature, from philosophy to poetry to medicine. I think I was always interested in autonomy growing up. I used to have to sit mute on my hospital bed as a swarm of white coats surrounded me, and my orthopaedic consultant would just take my leg affected with polio without asking, squeeze it, turn it and twist it in his examination. I was still attached it to it, remember. I would squirm, and sometimes yelp as it hurt, but I had no choice but to bear the ward rounds and the consultation, especially if I wanted my operations to go well. Back then, nearly 40 years ago, it was just what happened. Doctors told you what to do. Doctors knew best. And as a minor, I was lucky if I had any eye contact, let alone conversation. It didn't matter if I didn't like it. It didn't matter if I was in pain. I was helpless to stop it, and so I didn't. This experience affected me a lot, so much so that even years later, when I had a choice about a school project as an early teen, I wrote about the concept of autonomy. The importance of being able to choose your own death if you were in pain: autonomy in euthanasia. I never really understood 'autonomy' deeply until I studied philosophy at university, and I went on to study bioethics and law as a postgraduate. Interestingly, autonomy in mothers (with babies outside the womb) was never a concept we covered, and when I became a mother I understood why. Being autonomous in motherhood is different, as you are not only considering yourself in the equation, but another person with legal and moral rights that depends on you, and because of this you experience situations that put you under duress. A good example of this is a screaming hungry newborn: you are moved to act, your needs and your wants take second place, and you are no longer 'free' to do what you want. The duress causes you to act in a particular way. Nature designed it like this to ensure that small humans survive, by ensuring caregivers respond. I, like many others, found the struggle with being autonomous a challenge when becoming a mother, not only because of my habits of personal pursuit and my society's promotion of individualism, but also because I felt an incredible moral weight on my shoulders. I couldn't simply be an autonomous person anymore, as my actions affected another person so greatly. Was this the invisible weight of responsibility of keeping a little human alive? You could argue so, but I would say it deceptively wasn't: it was also the expectation of being 'a good mother'. To do 'mothering' well by ensuring I raised a good citizen who was unharmed by anything as a child – and to make sure I thoroughly enjoyed it as I went along. Rose's essay *Mothers: On Love and Cruelty* critiques how societies relentlessly blame mothers for the ills of the world through media and policies, and punish them for being anything but the ideal mother. At the heart of her argument is that mothers *will* fail, not that they do, not that they can, but that they will – and that it is okay.* It was a freeing notion for me, affirming the personal revolution against 'motherhood in modernity' I had felt welling up since I became a mother, and it gave me the permission I needed to write this book about breastfeeding in all its darkness, and glory. Permission to blame everything else but ourselves for aversion, permission to be frank about cause and consequence when breastfeeding in the 21st century. Permission to share the truths of mothers who felt like monsters, and the manifestation of the stresses and difficulties of life when breastfeeding. Because, I realised, if we leave out the darkness of aversion, and do not tell the stories of women who experience it, we are telling an untruth. Idealised motherhood and reality are rarely the same, and if we do not tell the story of how aversion can plague the life of breastfeeding mothers we are depriving mothers of the tools of expression they need to understand what is happening to them, and excluding them from a world they think does not exist, making them completely alone.

I am an advocate of 'forewarned is forearmed' with breastfeeding aversion, as I think it may lessen the risk of getting it, because expectations around breastfeeding can affect your emotions and how you respond to situations in reality. The difficulty of this forewarning is that explaining the entirety of all the possible experiences you may have as a breastfeeding mother is simply not possible in an antenatal class, and it isn't really covered by governmental health organisations or independent breastfeeding institutions. I know many organisations have shied away from addressing breastfeeding aversion for fear of scaring new mothers away from 'trying to breastfeed'. However, we are in a time of irrepressibility. No longer will women stay quiet when they are expected to: the 'mommy wars' are a testament to this.

The widely divisive choices mothers make are at once celebrated and criticised; there is no one 'right' way to mother anymore. With the world leaping forward through

---

*   Rose, J. (2018). *Mothers: An Essay on Love and Cruelty* (Main edition). London: Faber & Faber.

technological advances that have brought the internet and social media, social movements are now concentrating on minority rights, like those of mothers. But because in modern life everyone is right – as choice is king – you can have directly opposing movements. As a mother, you can choose to birth at home, or birth in hospital, breastfeed or formula feed, sleep train or respond at night, bed-share or put the baby in a separate room. Every decision is a 'right' decision, in that it's the individual's choice that matters, and, crucially, mothers should be happy that they can choose. But the National Institute for Mental Health report found that mental health issues were one of the main causes of disease burden worldwide,[*] and estimates of women who experience postnatal mood disorders, including anxiety and depression, are increasing.[**] Why? Well, in case it isn't clear by now, I think that one reason is that maternal instincts and a woman's ability to mother are being tampered with, diluted, and obstructed. The aspects of life that are ordinarily experienced in the journey of motherhood are intensified because of this tampering, and the difficulties that follow are like a 'domino effect' because sometimes only one step has been delayed, removed, or replaced. Take giving birth vaginally: what happens when you don't? You may be fine. Or you may struggle with infection or with recovery, you may struggle with bonding with your baby, getting baby to latch, and so struggle with breastfeeding. All of these have been shown to be affected by having major abdominal surgery, more commonly known as a 'C-section'. You may have birth trauma or breastfeeding trauma[***] and little postnatal support to help you come to terms with it, while at the same time expecting motherhood to be a certain way, and viewing yourself as a mother who has categorically

[*] *Fundamental-facts-about-mental-health-2016.pdf*. (n.d.). Retrieved from https://www.mentalhealth.org.uk/sites/default/files/fundamental-facts-about-mental-health-2016.pdf

[**] Field, T. (2018). Postnatal anxiety prevalence, predictors and effects on development: A narrative review. *Infant Behavior & Development, 51*, 24–32.

[***] Brown, A. (2019). *Why Breastfeeding Grief and Trauma Matter*. Pinter & Martin Ltd.

failed – even though everyone else around you is saying you didn't. All of these factors have been linked to postnatal mood disorders and depression.

Somehow, even if breastmilk is amazing, and breastfeeding is the best thing to do as a mother, does it matter if these statements do not acknowledge the truth of the experiential difficulty of mothering through breastfeeding in the 21st century, and that mothers will 'fail'? Aside from all the complex mothering relationships Rose covers in her book, from the absent mother, to the detached mother, to the adoring mother, for me there is one thing that ties them all together. We cannot mother alone, and we cannot mother in a responsive way as nature intended when we no longer live in a way that nature intended. I wonder, do we keep saying yes to breastfeeding our infants when we really mean no, because we are crippled by wanting to do best for them and not having an alternative choice of action? Certainly many mothers tell me this through their words:

> I am constantly battling my need to create space and respite from mothering with my guilt of not doing enough as a mum, I think that's why I can't stop breastfeeding. I just feel like it would harm them by weaning before they are ready.
> Natalia, Rio de Janeiro

The explosion of research into breastfeeding, breastmilk and infant development is often considered in a silo of limited variables and biological norms, without application to the society we live in now. I wonder how much we personally over-emphasise this information and apply it to our own lives, which are a different context. We need to breastfeed because we make milk after birth, because most of us want to breastfeed,[*] and because it is our main tool to get our nurslings to sleep, to console and comfort them, as we have seen in the concept

***

[*] Over 80% of women initiate breastfeeding in the UK, but less than 1% exclusively breastfeed by six months, found at the WBTi UK report published in Parliament in 2016. *Wbti-uk-report-2016-part-1-14-2-17. pdf.* (n.d.). Retrieved from ukbreastfeedingtrends.files.wordpress. com/2017/03/wbti-uk-report-2016-part-1-14-2-17.pdf

of nurture, and that is how nature intended it. However, we are no longer 'in nature'. Everything around us except the responsive breastfeeding is unnatural. Our artificial lights, our artificial food, our artificial construct of time, our artificial screens transporting us into a completely different world of fiction and fantasy . . . and then there is social media. This bizarre tiny other world in our phones results in very limited and often one-way communication with other sentient beings in real time, through an artificial interface that is spectacularly unnatural, leading to inauthentic and awkward interactions in the 'real world' with online people we know.

Many of us know about the importance of babies and children having secure attachment to their mother, and the importance of breastfeeding, but being so much more informed, unbeknownst to us, disempowers us when aversion strikes. We are too scared to do anything wrong for fear of harming our nurslings, to night wean, to wean or just to stop breastfeeding. And then there are the negative emotions, which are a heavy weight that many bear in silence. To speak openly about feelings of hate toward other adult human beings, let alone children, is unspeakable, if you'll excuse the pun. Yet the paediatrician Winnicott thought that infants learn to love only by learning to hate, and that they have to experience hate from the mother in order to do this.[*] This revolutionary opinion is one of the many missed bits of knowledge mothers don't have access to and are not exposed to. Then there is the generation gap that missed breastfeeding – formula in a bottle was the predominant method of feeding in the 1980s[**] – and the lack of mothering knowledge being passed down, which means many of us have no role models to show us *how* to set boundaries, or *how* to wean, and we have nothing to tell us that weaning at five months or five years will mean our nursling will be 'alright'. Many mothers need to stop breastfeeding in the middle of a session; they need a release, they need to execute their desire or need to do something, but they cannot. This then happens

---

[*] WINNICOTT, D. W. (1994). Hate in the Counter-Transference. *The Journal of Psychotherapy Practice and Research*, 3(4), 348–356.

[**] Stevens, E. E., Patrick, T. E., & Pickler, R. (2009). A History of Infant Feeding. *The Journal of Perinatal Education*, 18(2), 32–39.

again and again. This level of restriction and stress has to affect them in some way. And how a mother deals with stress will affect how they deal with stress *when* breastfeeding. With all the other stresses that being a mother brings, our subconscious creeps in, and negative thoughts arise.

These thoughts are things like: I had a *better* life than this, I have so many things I *could* be doing, this is not how motherhood *should* be. We become irritated as we repeat our 'story' and our frustrations in our head, and aversion strikes. Aversion for some mothers is the manifestation of an inability to reclaim their sense of autonomy, of control. To have the life you thought you would have, the one you feel you deserve. This loss of control can be extended to the desire to reclaim your body, because of feeling trapped in a breastfeeding session, or a breastfeeding relationship, which may be becoming overwhelming, and that we feel we cannot get out of. However, it seems here that aversion is only the end of the narrative. To further understand what is happening in mothers who get aversion we need to look not only at the current situation, but also at the beginning of their stories – what happened to them as children – and the middle part of their stories: who these women were before they were mothers.

Risk factors for developing aversion

Although we may not have the medical research to know the exact cause of aversion, we can be pretty confident that it is not something that happens randomly. As mothers themselves can sometimes attribute their triggers to difficulties they faced in the past, or how frustrated and run down they feel being a mother, it is important to consider all factors in a woman's life that could contribute to aversion, including from before she became a mother. Dr Gabor Maté has written and spoken extensively on the role of hidden stress in relation to health conditions, showing that there is a direct link between living in ways that create stress and associated poor health.[*] He makes a

---

[*]   Maté, G. (2019). *When the body says no: The cost of hidden stress*. Melbourne; Scribe.

strong case for many health conditions being 'biopsychosocial', with all three factors contributing to a person's health. This is in part why I wrote so much about modern-day society and lifestyle, how it can relate to breastfeeding, and why it should be considered in aversion. There are many risk factors that can play into experiencing aversion, including the mother's previous history, biological state, traumatic events past or present, as well as her current physical health and support structure. The phenomenon of aversion does have a demonstrable biopsychosocial nature to it, like many medical conditions, although I don't think aversion is necessarily a 'medical condition'. The link between upbringing, social environment and health conditions has been around for many years, with an overwhelming amount of research that has shown us the extent to which these conditions can affect an individual. Indices of deprivation and links to poor health are now used across public health to improve health outcomes. The Adverse Childhood Experiences study has shown without a doubt that experiencing certain traumas as a child affects lifelong health and opportunity. The effects of adverse childhood experiences have an impact on physical health, change behaviours and affect learning later in life. This study was a game-changer in preventative medicine and looked at the relationship between childhood abuse and household dysfunction on adult life by assessing ten key areas that children experienced, including having an absent parent, substance misuse, and all kinds of abuse. The authors found a strong and graded relationship of exposure to adverse childhood effects as well as risk factors for many of the leading causes of death in adults.[*] The general gist of the findings is that you cannot separate what happened to you as a child from who you are today, and you cannot separate who you are from how it affects your health. We know, for example, that most women who have experienced

---

[*]   Felitti, V. J., Anda, R. F., Nordenberg, D., Williamson, D. F., Spitz, A. M., Edwards, V., … Marks, J. S. (1998). Relationship of Childhood Abuse and Household Dysfunction to Many of the Leading Causes of Death in Adults: The Adverse Childhood Experiences (ACE) Study. *American Journal of Preventive Medicine, 14*(4), 245–258. https://doi. org/10.1016/S0749-3797(98)00017-8

childhood sexual abuse want to breastfeed, and do go on to try to breastfeed. We also know that being a survivor of childhood abuse is associated with an increase in the number of biologically associated breastfeeding problems like mastitis and pain.* There are direct links between what happens in our childhood and our breastfeeding experience and ability for some women.

Extensive research has also been conducted into prenatal exposure to stress. One recent study found that beliefs and expectations about breastfeeding, distress during pregnancy, and anxiety and depressive symptoms were associated with changes in breastfeeding initiation and continuation. The authors posit that assessing and addressing pre- and postnatal distress could improve breastfeeding rates.** The stress of mothers is a factor for the stress of infants, and ultimately infant exposure to stress. The early formative years are known to be a time of particular vulnerability if experiencing early adversity, because the brain and other organ systems are undergoing dramatic changes as they develop, grow rapidly and mature. A study published in 2019 by Pierce and colleagues found that particular effects of caregiver stress and maternal educational level on the neurodevelopment of an infant are detectable even as young as two months of life.***

A life event that happened many years ago may seem irrelevant when thinking about what can help with aversion, but on closer consideration you can see that childhood adversity, previous sexual abuse, or even something recent like birth trauma are not only interlinked, but can be shown to

---

* Elfgen, C., Hagenbuch, N., Görres, G., Block, E., & Leeners, B. (2017). Breastfeeding in Women Having Experienced Childhood Sexual Abuse: *Journal of Human Lactation*. https://doi.org/10.1177/0890334416680789
** Ritchie-Ewing, G., Mitchell, A. M., & Christian, L. M. (2019). Associations of Maternal Beliefs and Distress in Pregnancy and Postpartum With Breastfeeding Initiation and Early Cessation. *Journal of Human Lactation*, 35(1), 49–58. https://doi.org/10.1177/0890334418767832
*** Pierce, L. J., Thompson, B. L., Gharib, A., Schlueter, L., Reilly, E., Valdes, V., … Nelson, C. A. (2019). Association of Perceived Maternal Stress During the Perinatal Period With Electroencephalography Patterns in 2-Month-Old Infants. *JAMA Pediatrics*, 173(6), 561–570.

contribute to negative emotions. Observations about the way women link the constraint of breastfeeding with the weight and burden of motherhood, coupled with current pressures, show underlying causes for their struggles with negative emotions linked to the activity of breastfeeding. For some years now I have run a structured support course online, as well as a peer-to-peer support group. I have seen that there are certain circumstances in which mothers experience aversion, perhaps due to the nature of the challenges they can create in her life. I also see particular characteristics in a mother and nursling, and have concluded that there are a few categories that could mean a mother is at risk of developing aversion. Identifying possible risk factors for aversion will help mothers, as it will tell us about what the root cause may be, and more about what needs to be done to lessen or remove aversion. From the current metadata we have, the following areas repeatedly come when in supporting women with aversion:

Physical

- Breastfeeding difficulties, for example with a premature baby, or a baby that doesn't latch to the breast. Aversion may not strike while experiencing the difficulty, but further down the line when a negative association with breastfeeding has been developed.
- Persistent nipple or breast pain, and discomfort when breastfeeding. This could be feeding with a restrictive tongue-tie, persistent nipple contact with the palate, Raynaud's syndrome, repeated cases of mastitis or thrush, or unexplained pain.
- Breastfeeding during pregnancy with a reduction of supply, dry feeding and bodily changes including sensitive nipples.

Dyad- or 'pair'-specific

- Tandem breastfeeding either when pregnant and breastfeeding, or feeding a newborn and an older child.
- Breastfeeding twins or multiples.
- Breastfeeding an older child (particularly when teething,

with a poor latch, or constant movement, when aversion is a natural biological trigger to wean off the breast).

- Mother's sensitivity to stressors (including physical, sensory, auditory etc).

Biological

- The return of postnatal menses, monthly menstruation, and monthly ovulation.
- Lack of sleep, disturbed sleep or inability to return to sleep after breastfeeding at night.
- Inadequate nutrition and poor hydration.

Psychological

- Survivor of previous or childhood sexual abuse.
- Social or external pressures on the mother's time, including external work or educational deadlines, the return to work, and caregiving for other children.
- Birth or previous breastfeeding trauma.

Medical factors

- Adverse childhood experiences, early childhood trauma, or recent trauma.
- Dysphoric Milk Ejection Reflex (D-MER).
- Clinical depression.
- Postnatal depression and anxiety.
- Gender dysphoria.*

With the challenges that arise from these particular experiences, there is more likelihood that negative emotions at the breast will be triggered – particularly if aversion is not

---

* I have not extensively supported transgender persons through aversion and this is not my specialist area, nor is this book aimed at the LBGT community as I have primarily researched breastfeeding mothers. However, people struggling with gender dysphoria who are breastfeeding or chest-feeding can and do experience varying levels of aversion, and I believe are at risk of experiencing for some of the same reasons as women, like loss of control and reduced body autonomy. But also distinctly due to body and hormonal changes that come with pregnancy and lactation.

etiologically hormonal, or due to a specific recent event in a mother's life. Variations in a mother's ability to respond to adversity will mean there are variations in the way mothers are able to cope with breastfeeding challenges, and in how breastfeeding restriction affects them. One mother's prison is another mother's heaven, and all the will in the world cannot change how it is perceived or experienced unless you know why it is happening. Having positive emotions and feelings when breastfeeding, having oxytocin working properly and having a positive association with breastfeeding will mean that being stuck in a dark room alone at night isn't the worst thing in the world: you are in love with your nursling, and it could even be nice! The exact opposite situation will mean an enormous mental and emotional struggle, which takes its toll on your mental health; you feel stuck like a prisoner, against your will. Furthermore, humans will strive to exercise their autonomy for survival: as much as we need social interaction to survive, we also need a certain amount of personal space and freedom for our sanity. Mothers with nurslings have very real restrictions, which makes this freedom rather more complicated to achieve. The list of risk factors for aversion can give us an idea of whether you are more likely to develop it. But these risk factors also indicate where the negative sensations and negative responses of aversion may occur. The more they occur, the more likely they are to become part of the breastfeeding journey due to the vicious aversion cycle, and the more severe the aversion will become over time if the root problem or the situational and personal triggers are not resolved.

Relief from pain and discomfort

Pain and discomfort in the early days of breastfeeding are in many ways normal, so the idea that 'breastfeeding doesn't hurt' is simply false. When you are a new mother breastfeeding for the first time your nipples can feel uncomfortable as they are pulled out, and also if your nursling is tiny compared to the size of your breast and nipple, and they struggle to open wide. Three days – or three weeks – of this can seem an eternity of pain. Getting used to latching may cause redness and tenderness on nipple when the attachment isn't optimal. Women can then experience soreness and tenderness with engorgement as the milk 'comes in', and many experience an intense tingling when their milk flows at the beginning of a feed. Then there is the stomach tightening that comes when breastfeeding, which many women complain is 'as painful as labour contractions', as the womb returns to its normal size. Newborn feeding patterns can lead to more engorgement, which makes the breasts feel hot, heavy, extremely sensitive to touch, uncomfortable and painful. Although these sensations ease when nurslings suckle and milk is removed, women can also experience blocked ducts and mastitis, which can be incredibly painful. And this pain is just a few days or weeks into breastfeeding. We can consider this pain normal in a way – a temporary set of pain experiences if you will – as these problems will usually resolve themselves for many mothers.

Persistent or severe pain, however, though we know it occurs, is almost always a sign that something isn't quite right. Pain is one major factor that can interfere with breastfeeding and it is known that mothers will wean earlier than they want to because of nipple or breast pain, but there is little research about the intensity or type of pain. Many women with aversion continue to breastfeed through persistent pain or discomfort. It is not clear why some stop and others continue.

Having nipple pain when breastfeeding can happen with or without any visible trauma, and you can experience persistent nipple pain despite having had successful treatment for nipple lesions or breast infections.* The authors of one study on pain in breastfeeding concluded that the ramifications of nipple pain extend far beyond the act of breastfeeding, particularly for women whose pain lasts several months. Even after accounting for pain intensity they found a greater interference with mood, sleep and even general activity was linked to

---

* McClellan, H.L., Hepworth, A.R., Garbin, C.P., Rowan, M.K., Deacon, J., Hartmann, P.E., & Geddes, D.T. (2012). Nipple Pain during Breast-feeding with or without Visible Trauma. *Journal of Human Lactation*, *28*(4), 511–521.

having a longer duration of nipple pain.* Pain, whether acute or chronic, can and does affect women, and their emotions, when they are breastfeeding. And many women continue to breastfeed despite pain, which is why, in addition to my earlier argument for pain being one clear cause of aversion, I believe it is also a risk factor for aversion:

> *My twins have small mouths and terrible latches, I used to dread every feed as I would sometimes get so angry at their inefficiency (irrational I know as they weren't doing it on purpose!!). So many tears and so much anguish meant I threw in the towel at six months and to be honest it was a huge relief as the massive psychological burden of it all was threatening to drag me under.* Nemani, Bangalore

Depression

I came from a broken home, where my father was a perpetrator of domestic violence. I contracted polio from a vaccination and lived around half my childhood as in inpatient in a large orthopaedic hospital. Back then, after surgery, you would stay on a ward to recover, and after each of my operations this would take anywhere from six to eight months. Through these experiences I have learned there are few definitive answers in life about why things happen and what to do about them. Whether it be questions about your childhood, your lot in life, or your health: there is always more than one way to look at things. I found this also applies to the field of medicine. When it came to my recent medical diagnosis of post-polio syndrome, I found that different doctors had opposing views about what I had for many years. Lately, when scouring journals and devouring books to research this one, it has become clear that doctors and counsellors also disagree about the causes of depression, and how to treat it. Disconnection from your emotions and 'dis-ease' in your life can now be diagnosed as a medical condition with a chemical imbalance as the cause, but as Hilary Hendel writes and practises: 'It's

---

*   Ibid.

Not Always Depression"*. However, in saying this it is still important to consider what is now normatively understood as depression, and what the symptoms of depression are in relation to aversion, as there are crossovers. When we covered oxytocin's role in aversion and the links to the social nervous system, we considered the fight or flight response in breastfeeding mothers. The fight or flight behaviour is also common in depression, and as people do not tend to flee life situations any longer (generally there are no bears attacking us), people who are depressed can become aggressive – which could be one interpretation of the negative emotion of anger or agitation with aversion. Also, people often do not recognise that they have fallen into depression, and this may be the case for mothers too, so I want to be sure to give depression its due when we look at what aversion is. Understanding it may be key for you, or the mothers you support.

According to the World Health Organization, mental health illnesses and depression will be the second most prevalent global burden of disease by 2020, after heart disease." Some do not consider it a disease in an etiological sense, but an appropriate and normal response to an impossible or intolerable situation. Depression after loss of a loved one is one example of this. Other recent research has shown that stress can trigger an inflammation process that can lead to depression,*** and some even believe that inflammation is not simply *a* risk factor for depression but *the* risk factor, because it underpins all the other risk factors.**** New research by Robles and colleagues in the theory of stress causing an inflammatory response suggests that all types of stress,

*   Hendel, H.J. (2018a). *It's Not Always Depression: A New Theory of Listening to Your Body, Discovering Core Emotions and Reconnecting with Your Authentic Self.* Penguin Life.
**   Kessler, R.C., & Bromet, E.J. (2013). The epidemiology of depression across cultures. *Annual Review of Public Health, 34,* 119–138.
***   Kendall-Tackett, K. (2010b). Four Research Findings That Will Change What We Think About Perinatal Depression. *Journal of Perinatal Education, 19*(4), 7–9.
****Berk, M., Williams, L.J., Jacka, F.N., O'Neil, A., Pasco, J.A., Moylan, S., ... Maes, M. (2013). So depression is an inflammatory disease, but where does the inflammation come from? *BMC Medicine, 11*(1), 200.

including psychological and physical, can lead to depression.[*] Postnatal depression, anxiety and mood disorders are common all around the world and on the rise, so it would be unwise not to consider them in the phenomenon of aversion. Depression can manifest in a spectrum of emotions, including anger and irritation – like aversion – so it's only natural to ask, is aversion actually depression? I wouldn't rule out them being one and the same in some mothers, but not others. Ultimately, it would be a matter for a healthcare practitioner who is knowledgeable about maternal mental health and infant feeding to screen and properly assess a mother. Research will tell us more in time, but for now we have to be able to help ourselves and improve our situation.

We know that the symptoms of depression do not necessarily stay the same throughout the period of depression, and that they are not uniform among a population, although they can include anxiety, suicidal tendencies and self-harm. In general, these seem to be different from the symptoms of aversion, which include anger and agitation triggered by activity at the breast, and intrusive thoughts about getting free or pushing the child off. With depression there are usually other psychological symptoms like feelings of irritability, low mood, sadness, helplessness, tearfulness, and guilt. Depression is also known by its physical symptoms, which can include an increase or decrease in appetite and consequently weight, unexplained aches or pains, lack of libido, lack of energy, constipation, changes in the menstrual cycle, sleep disturbance and speaking more slowly than usual. If you struggled with depression before becoming a mother, or if you had a traumatic birth, you are more likely to experience postnatal depression, which we know can affect breastfeeding. While research shows breastfeeding can serve to *protect* you from depression, if it is not going well it can actually be a risk factor for *getting* depression. So, having challenges with breastfeeding will mean you are more likely

---

[*]   Robles, T.F., Glaser, R., & Kiecolt-Glaser, J.K. (2005). Out of Balance: A New Look at Chronic Stress, Depression, and Immunity. *Current Directions in Psychological Science*, *14*(2), 111–115.

to develop postnatal depression, and I think that these both play into experiencing aversion. This is because breastfeeding challenges and difficulties usually mean experiencing pain, consequent stress and subsequent emotional turbulence. And because inflammation comes hand-in-hand with pain and stress.[*][**] Pain, stress and emotional imbalances are a perfect breeding ground for aversion. I would also argue that being depressed may mean you are more likely to get aversion, because of the challenges depression can bring to decision-making and coping with stressful situations.

There is no clinical evidence at present to indicate that aversion is postnatal depression, although some of the presenting symptoms may lead the mother, or even healthcare practitioners, to conclude this. Anger, agitation, disgust, guilt, and shame, alongside intrusive thoughts, could easily be diagnosed as depression, especially if the mother presenting to a doctor has a newborn baby. A doctor may naturally assume postnatal depression, given its prevalence and the similarity of symptoms. But this does not necessarily make sense for mothers of toddlers or older nurslings. And many women are surprised when they experience aversion, as they have had a previously wonderful breastfeeding relationship, often saying 'it came out of nowhere'.[***] It's a difficult and sensitive area, as some mothers may not actually know they are depressed, especially if the depression develops over time. As a general rule, feeling persistently hopeless and losing interest in life and the things that you enjoy are clear signs that you may be struggling with depression, rather than experiencing negative emotions when breastfeeding. You can have depression for weeks, months or years and it can be mild, moderate or severe. It is well known that depression can affect your work, social and home life, causing difficulties and imbalance in all of those

---

*   Ibid.
**   Kendall-Tackett, K. (2010b). Four Research Findings That Will Change What We Think About Perinatal Depression. *Journal of Perinatal Education*, *19*(4), 7–9.
***   Once you take the screening questions and have an in-depth assessment, a skilled doctor who should be able to decipher if you have clinical depression, or not.

areas. For mothers, the postnatal period is a common time for depression to strike, so if you are unsure about whether your aversion is really depression it would be best to seek medical advice. If you really are only affected with negative emotions when breastfeeding, and have a number of the symptoms listed, then it is unlikely that you are depressed, especially if you are generally feeling okay and enjoying other areas of your life. As a mother told me: 'I am not depressed, but I find breastfeeding depressing'.

A similar evaluation should happen when considering postnatal anxiety. Anxiety and depression are two separate but often interconnected conditions. They are considered in the medical community as 'comorbid', which means they are often found together. Anxiety is important to consider in aversion because it is a response to information we have gathered that we register as a threat. According to Goleman, we can buffer ourselves from anxiety when we use our attention to deny a threat,* and this is important when looking at what happens when aversion strikes.

Anxiety

Anxiety is an emotional state that many people find unpleasant, which includes having feelings of uneasiness, fear, and even excitement. Paul and colleagues found that the immediate changes in our roles and responsibilities in life straight after childbirth can provoke anxiety.** Postnatal anxiety is more prevalent than postnatal depression, but prolonged anxiety is thought to increase the risk of postnatal depression, so it is important to consider it when we look at the biopsychosocial model of the phenomenon of aversion. While anxiety is a normal response and part of the human assessment and survival process, how it affects mothers varies. A study by Horsely and colleagues in 2019 found that pregnancy-

* Goleman, D. (1998). *Vital Lies, Simple Truths: The Psychology of Self-deception* (New edition edition). London: Bloomsbury Publishing PLC
** Paul, I.M., Downs, D.S., Schaefer, E.W., Beiler, J.S.B., & Weisman, C.S. (2013). Postpartum anxiety and maternal-infant health outcomes. *Pediatrics, 131*(4), NaN-NaN.

specific anxiety was associated with lower odds of exclusive breastfeeding at the six to eight week period after birth for some mothers.[*] Anxiety is directly relevant when looking at risk factors for aversion because of how it affects breastfeeding. A normal level of maternal anxiety about a newborn provides the heightened state of alertness needed to ensure the needs of a baby are met, and that any dangers to a vulnerable baby are eradicated. In the early days this can mean being 'on guard' 24 hours a day. Babies need to be fed, and cared for day and night, so even when babies are asleep mothers often report 'checking that they are still breathing', which I am sure some of you remember. In essence, you are never 'off duty'. This heightened awareness and intense care gradually declines as the infant becomes more independent: more able to move their body, to take intended actions, and then to verbalise their needs. However, many mothers find that the experience of intensive care doesn't decline, and anxiety levels stay high as a nursling's needs and temperament change unpredictably (typically with perceived sleep 'regressions' and developmental changes).

What happens when this kind of normal, healthy level of anxiety found at the beginning of newborn care doesn't subside? Using Goleman's understanding of anxiety, our 'attention-gathering-skills' become skewed and we do not or cannot cushion ourselves from anxiety. A typical scene for mothers may be a sleepless night, lying breastfeeding in a dark room. Imagine you are trying to sleep, but instead you are thinking about where you have to be tomorrow morning at 9am sharp, how tired you already are, when your baby will wake up next, and also all the things you have to do this year! You start to feel a bit warm, and you can feel your heart pumping a little harder. You try to smile and brush it off, to stop thinking about everything and *just relax*. The bed is warm; your baby is okay. Yes, your head hurts, your eyes sting and you feel bloated from eating rubbish food today, but you know that all that disappears once you have had some sleep. You

* Horsley, K., Nguyen, T.-V., Ditto, B., & Da Costa, D. (2019). The Association Between Pregnancy-Specific Anxiety and Exclusive Breastfeeding Status Early in the Postpartum Period. *Journal of Human Lactation*, 0890334419838482.

turn to get comfortable, and all the thoughts come flooding back. Your heart beats a little faster now, and again you try to curb your anxiety. You reach for your phone to divert your attention for a while. This cycle repeats for the next hour. Now you're starting to get frustrated, and you can't fall asleep even though you know you have to. You're wondering whether it is worth it anymore, as your baby will probably wake in less than half an hour to feed again. Having to wake up when you have finally fallen asleep will make you feel even worse than if you had just stayed awake – and you run the risk of not being able to get back to sleep again afterwards too. This scenario explains a situation in which anxiety can be very severe. Even when you lie in the dark and do nothing, trying to relax, or to 'breathe it out', it can be very difficult to stop your body from doing what it's doing: reacting to the build-up of internal mental stress by skewing the information gathered.

This description of a night isn't a one-off for some mothers; it is a frequent, even nightly occurrence. Never being able to catch up on sleep, and always being on overdrive, means they are always overtired, which then feeds into the cycle of adrenaline and cortisol release and subsequently not being able to fall asleep easily to get the restorative sleep they so desperately need. Add another child into the mix, and it becomes more complex and the mother becomes more frustrated, sleep-deprived and powerless. Carry this on for a few years and it becomes a chronic situation. Cognitive decision-making wanes, food choices lean toward the high in sugar and high in fat, and you become at risk of lots of health conditions. And all the while this mother is responsible for the lives of her children, as well as the pseudo-responsibilities of modern life, like 'showing up', 'looking good', and 'doing stuff' every day with your children to 'be a good mother'. The impact of severe sleep deprivation and its relation to anxiety is not to be discounted. Sleep deprivation is the perfect breeding ground for negative thoughts, where the 'normal' seeds of anxiety can grow like weeds and consume a mother.

Depression and anxiety are serious conditions that have specific descriptions and a cluster of symptoms. Both can leave you in a more difficult situation as a mother, making coping with restricting and emotionally challenging breastfeeding situations, like persistent pain, the despair of night-time feeding, or the negotiation of weaning, even harder. They can make having aversion more likely, but it is important to differentiate aversion from depression and anxiety for other clinical reasons. Conditions that have overlapping mechanisms or causes, like stress, need to be considered in order to specifically address aversion, especially when taking antidepressants or counselling for depression do not work, because aversion seems to be related to breastfeeding-specific activities. Being diagnosed with depression when you present to a doctor with aversion, and being prescribed a treatment drug to improve your condition, may not work if you are in persistent pain or being triggered when breastfeeding from a traumatic event in your past.

Dysphoric Milk Ejection Reflex (D-MER)

This process of diagnosing the right condition is important to consider when aversion is similar to other conditions such as D-MER, in which women experience feelings of dysphoria during the let-down that dissipate after the let-down finishes. Aversion is similar in that feelings of dysphoria would generally be considered to be 'negative' feelings, and perhaps a signal or message that something is wrong. Aversion is also similar in that some women will have to self-harm in order to 'see out' the feed, ie, not to prematurely de-latch. Pinching themselves, biting down on their hand or holding their breast very tightly to the point of cutting off the blood supply are all coping actions that mothers describe when they have aversion or D-MER and are trying to 'get through a feed'. Nonetheless, healthcare practitioners and doctors, whose business it is to differentiate similar symptoms to understand and diagnose specific conditions, recognise that there are some very clear differences between the two. For example, different negative emotions, different causal mechanisms and different durations. Whereas D-MER is thought to be a medical condition with a clear hormonal cause, aversion is not, but I do know that aversion can be experienced by women who have D-MER, and that women can differentiate between the two.

There are many crossovers in the difficulties mothers with aversion and mothers with D-MER face, and stress seems to be a player in both. Ruglass and Kendall-Tackett argue that the symptomatic patterns of women struggling with D-MER are like those found in people with post-traumatic stress disorder, who have chronic hyperarousal symptoms, meaning that they are always looking out for danger because their stress systems are always 'online' so to speak.[*] This is because D-MER is thought by some to be a short-term stress response triggered by oxytocin.[**] The negative feelings in D-MER are triggered in a part of the brain that is not within the mother's conscious control. These subconscious defensive reactions are there for mothers to protect their babies when necessary, but it seems with D-MER that they are triggered inappropriately because there is no actual danger. Moberg believes that the burst of oxytocin mistakenly activates the mother's defence reactions, rather than the more normal positive feelings that are associated with breastfeeding.[***] The short-term stress response that can be linked to maternal aggression is also seen in aversion. I would argue that aversion is causally associated with D-MER, but not the other way around. So experiencing aversion does not mean you will experience D-MER, but experiencing D-MER may mean you are likely to experience aversion, due to the added challenges and emotional burden when breastfeeding.

Previous sexual abuse

Although the number varies from country to country, about one in four women, or 20–25 percent, suffer from

[*]   Kendall-Tackett, K. A., & Ruglass, L. M. (2017). *Women's Mental Health Across the Lifespan: Challenges, Vulnerabilities, and Strengths.* Taylor & Francis.
[**] Uvnäs-Moberg, K., & Kendall-Tackett, K. (2018). The Mystery of D-MER: What Can Hormonal Research Tell Us About Dysphoric Milk-Ejection Reflex? *Clinical Lactation, 9*(1), 23–29.
[***] Ibid

sexual trauma,[*] and there are rising rates of childhood sexual abuse around the world.[**] Being a survivor of sexual abuse can affect people in different ways. While some people can function normally as adults, others will have various symptoms as a result of their abuse, which can be both physical and psychological.[***] It is common to have adult manifestations of a chronic response to experiencing childhood abuse. Stressful life events like birth, death, marriage and divorce can trigger the return of the symptoms of childhood abuse. This phenomenon is called *sequela* and is a pathological condition that arises or results from disease, trauma or injury. Symptoms can include, but are not limited to: emotional reactions, negative emotions of shame, guilt, fear and humiliation, symptoms of post-traumatic stress, and distorted self-perception.[****] The underlying themes of body autonomy and consent in struggling with aversion are no more apparent than when you have experienced abuse:

I have been sexually abused as a child and as an adult was trapped in an abusive relationship where I was repeatedly and systematically raped and sexually humiliated . . . I have managed to breastfeed up until now with only short bouts of aversion but my little person is not as little anymore and has started furiously fighting to latch when I'm 'touched out', sore, have just been bitten or half asleep, etc. I ask them to stop but my little one is very wilful and has become quite forceful . . . they lift my top up, grab at my breasts and nipples with ferocity . . . I understand that there is no malice in their

* What Is the Impact of Sexual Trauma on Breastfeeding (2017, August 17). Retrieved 30 April 2019, from Women's Health Today website: https://womenshealthtoday.blog/2017/08/17/what-is-the-impact-of-sexual-trauma-on-breastfeeding/
** Child sexual abuse and exploitation: UN event sheds light on the unthinkable. (2018, October 3). Retrieved 22 October 2019, from UN News website: https://news.un.org/en/story/2018/10/1022152
*** Adult Manifestations of Childhood Sexual Abuse—ACOG. (n.d.). Retrieved 8 September 2019: https://www.acog.org/Clinical-Guidance-and-Publications/Committee-Opinions/Committee-on-Health-Care-for-Underserved-Women/Adult-Manifestations-of-Childhood-Sexual-Abuse
****Ibid

thinking, they are just trying to get to their favourite food source, but I find this behaviour mega triggering. I know this isn't about my little one, it's about my past and my trauma.
Melanie, Diss

Kendall-Tackett describes seven common areas where the effects of childhood sexual abuse could affect breastfeeding for a mother including experiencing emotional distress, an impaired sense of self and even post-traumatic stress disorder.[*] For women who register the experience of motherhood as a threat because of the way their minds and bodies gather attention, breastfeeding and body contact can be a constant trigger.[**] We know that birth and breastfeeding can be traumatic, and despite having the intention, will and determination to breastfeed, birth and breastfeeding can be triggers for many survivors. The way older nurslings behave around the breast can also be a trigger for many women, especially as some nurslings can be demanding, aggressive and forceful in their requests for milk. It can be hard for mothers to accept that they become upset when their nurslings are breastfeeding. Mothers can rationalise that it is not the nursling's fault, but at the same time the feelings are not unwarranted, given her history. This mother explains how she is triggered based on her past abuse:

I hated being touched in the dark. While the early morning hours are hard for any new parent, they presented a unique challenge that I only recognised later. Sometimes, I would wake up to my baby's nails scratching at my skin. The revulsion I felt was extreme. I kept a small light on throughout the night to prevent waking up in total darkness, which led me to confusion and then panic. I had a mantra to remind myself, I was saying things like 'I am safe' and 'this is my baby.' Polema, Prague

---

[*] Kendall-Tackett, K. (1998). Breastfeeding and the Sexual Abuse Survivor. *Journal of Human Lactation*, 14(2), 125–130.

[**] See Goleman, D. (1998). *Vital Lies, Simple Truths: The Psychology of Self-deception* for a detailed thesis of 'Attention' being the gathering of information crucial to existence and 'Anxiety' as the response when that information registers as a threat.

As with aversion, the use of skin-to-skin as an intervention to improve the breastfeeding relationship should be assessed carefully for those with a history of previous sexual abuse and trauma because it can be very triggering.* Memory flashbacks are stored in the body and there may be an unconscious response as the fight or flight mode kicks in. Even if the danger is *perceived* – and there is no danger in reality – the body will still react to a situation. The amygdala is responsible for stimulating the fight or flight reaction in the body: it is there to alert us to danger. This is the body's internal mechanism for protection and survival and, on a biological level, it is often not in our control. In a normal situation all the sensations associated with a dangerous or stressful experience are processed by the amygdala and form sensory memory, which is then given to the hippocampus and in turn to the neocortex where it is stored, as a verbal or narrative memory. But being triggered repeatedly will make it more ingrained, because what happens in a dangerous or life-threatening situation is that there is a rapid influx of information, and all the sensory memories stay in the amygdala. It becomes trapped there, unable to be properly processed and stored by the neocortex – the region that helps us make sense of events and experiences – so past memories and current breastfeeding experiences can essentially overlap:

> *I was emotionally forced into sex and humiliated by my son's father. My son is the spitting image of his father and I know it's not the baby's fault. There is no malice there at all but when he's demanding the breast it can be very traumatic for me. I didn't admit my feelings and things got so bad that my sister-in-law had to take baby away for a week because I couldn't separate the past trauma from my son's actions.* Ida, Helsinki

Aversion is more likely to strike given the particular circumstances of these mothers, and in this sense it is a clear

---

* Uvnäs-Moberg, K., & Kendall-Tackett, K. (2018). The Mystery of D-MER: What Can Hormonal Research Tell Us About Dysphoric Milk-Ejection Reflex? *Clinical Lactation*, 9(1), 23–29.

risk factor. Setting boundaries and getting yourself back to a feeling of being in control can help, but mothers often do not give themselves permission to do what works for them and their families. Comparing themselves to other mothers is common, but those other mothers may not have the same past, nor the same triggers. Expressing milk and bottle-feeding, covering up your skin, and using affirmations to reaffirm your intention to breastfeed help some women get back 'in control' by reconfiguring their experience once they have understood the cause of their triggers:

> *Triggers are horrendous, I felt something awful when my clothes were pulled at, I found the best way for me was to keep saying and feeling – 'this is a new memory'. Creating good memories and good experiences to overwrite the bad ones. Rewriting my feelings to eliminate the association with the bad memory of my abuse. Breathing deeply to enhance calm, smiling to release positive brain chemicals, and relaxing. Knowing I am nurturing, I am loving. I am making a safe place; I am doing something beautiful. So now my mind doesn't trigger as much at all because I am in control, I am giving consent to my child to do this, I am loved, needed and want to do it.* Carly, Swansea

Pregnancy and tandem feeding

Flower states that pregnancy is a common time for breastfeeding agitation for about a quarter of mothers who breastfeed through pregnancy,[*] and others suggest that the negative feelings are due to pregnancy making the body think it is time to wean.[**] Sore breasts are common when breastfeeding during pregnancy, with as many as 74 percent of mothers experiencing really severe discomfort and even excruciating pain.[***]

---

[*] Flower, H., & O'Mara, P. (2003a). *Adventures in Tandem Nursing: Breastfeeding During Pregnancy and Beyond.* Schaumburg, Ill: La Leche League International, p47.

[**] Moscone, S. R., & Moore, M. J. (1993). Breastfeeding during pregnancy. *Journal of Human Lactation: Official Journal of International Lactation Consultant Association, 9*(2), 83–88.

[***] Newton N, Theotokatos M. 1979. Breastfeeding during pregnancy in

I think breastfeeding through pregnancy was one of the worst experiences of my life, I had never thought I would but my boy didn't want to stop and he was still so young I couldn't bear to wean him. I cannot describe to you the pain I felt when he was on, the aversion was horrific, I will never forgive myself. Zaria, Manchester

In the acclaimed series *Blue Planet,* David Attenborough explains that one reason twins are so rarely found in the wild is a lack of food and nutrient resources for milk-making mammals. He implies that monkeys who are well fed in a particular part of India where the specific species is revered, had twins that survived because of abundant and calorific milk for both nurslings. While we know mothers can make milk for two or more infants, how a mother sustains her calorific and mental energy is also a factor in being able to continue breastfeeding. These may not affect the quality of the milk you produce, but this doesn't mean they do not affect your mood, comfort or ability to continue breastfeeding. Tandem breastfeeding two or more nurslings is a common time for aversion to strike and is a risk factor specifically when breastfeeding two *simultaneously*:

I had it [aversion] when I was tandem feeding my twins when they were tiny. I have very sensitive nipples (!) and they also both had tongue-tie, which didn't help. I found it overwhelming and intense, felt queasy, and had restless legs. I used to read a book, look at my phone, watch TV etc to distract myself which helped a bit. Never had it when feeding them singly. I ended up taking a break from tandem feeding from about 12 weeks. I went back to it when they were five months and their latches were much better and the aversion was mainly gone unless I was very tired. Gill, Rugby

Although it seems that mothers who tandem feed or nurse multiples can get aversion for a combination of reasons, stopping tandem feeding often resolves it for a time:

503 women. In *Emotion and Reproduction.* London, England: Academic Press, 845-49.

After about six weeks I hated tandem feeding with a passion!! Didn't have any aversion when feeding singularly so that's what we did. Not period-related for me as only got it back when the twins were one. I just felt so overwhelmed and like a milk machine. Mary, Illinois

When we think of the factors we considered in the chapter 'Conflict and Preferences', from individual preferences and conditional breastfeeds to body sensitivity when pregnant, we can see a pathway for aversion to arise in these mothers, because all these factors are doubled when feeding multiple nurslings. And when we consider breastfeeding through pregnancy, we have an internal change in state that can affect a woman, with progressive body functions being directed toward growing a new human. These, to me, create new stressors around breastfeeding and body contact for some women, so breastfeeding while carrying a fetus becomes a risk factor for developing aversion. Many women want to continue to breastfeed, but find that they simply cannot as they did before becoming pregnant. And when considerations of weaning come into the picture, the situation can be more tense. Night weaning is often the first step that happens, simply out of exhaustion and because aversion becomes so severe at night. But weaning takes time, energy and consistency in order to work in a smooth way and can present a problem for a tired pregnant mother, or an already tired mother breastfeeding more than one nursling at night. There is also often a desire to fully wean off the breast during pregnancy, as the mother's physical and mental health needs outweigh her ability to respond to her current nursling, depending on how often feeds are requested, whether her milk has completely dried up, how painful she finds feeds and how well she is coping with her pregnancy. Weaning completely will also depend on whether she experiences aversion, and how severe it is. I would not be surprised if future research reveals that the majority of mothers who continue to feed throughout their entire pregnancy do not experience severe or lasting aversion, and that those who do have aversion have nurslings who are extremely reluctant to wean.

Self-assessment, non-disclosure and misdiagnosis

Oh itchy latched child,
why does it feel so gross when
it should feel like love
Nursing aversion haiku by Jane Kirby

Self-assessment

Now that we have identified some groups of mothers who may be at risk of developing aversion, I wanted to write a little about the process of self-assessment that appears to happen in the support groups online as mothers struggle with the experience of aversion and the lack of information available about what is happening to them. Aversion is an unacknowledged experience in medical literature, and this leads to two problems: first, non-disclosure to healthcare professionals, and second, misdiagnosis by healthcare professionals if symptoms are disclosed.

Non-disclosure

Aversion is not widely known about, and many breastfeeding women are not able to disclose that they are experiencing it. Many think that it is 'just them' and hide it, and many don't know it exists and therefore would not think to disclose it. Imagery and literature about breastfeeding do not acknowledge that breastfeeding can trigger negative emotions, which perpetuates the myth that only positive experiences and emotions are felt when breastfeeding. This leads many mothers to think and feel as though positive experiences and emotions are what they *ought* to have when breastfeeding. Some cognitive models of depression[*] argue that core beliefs a person holds result in what are known as *conditional assumptions,* self-imposed rules that protect the person against distress, which lead to a certain kind of behaviour that can be activated in specific situations. With the phenomenon

---

[*] Beck, A. T., & Dozois, D. J. A. (2011). Cognitive therapy: Current status and future directions. *Annual Review of Medicine, 62,* 397–409.

of aversion for example, a view or belief that breastfeeding should be enjoyable and foster a loving relationship might lead the mother to believe that she ought to hide emotions like anger and agitation when breastfeeding because it is abnormal or could mean they are excluded from a group. In short, if I hide the fact I get angry when I breastfeed then I will be included in the breastfeeding community. Metadata certainly suggests that this behaviour happens in women with aversion, and that there is real anxiety and apprehension about disclosing breastfeeding triggering negative feelings to peers, family, friends and healthcare professionals. Disclosure anxiety arises due to fear of not being believed, not being taken seriously, being told there must be something 'wrong with them' as a mother by their partners, or being told they are postnatally depressed by healthcare professionals. These are all reasons that women who experience aversion and who are apprehensive about disclosing have reported.

Misdiagnosis

There are those who brave the reactions and reach out to tell others of their feelings and what is happening to them. Women who experience aversion who do disclose to their doctor have been told that they 'must be postnatally depressed'. Many women contest this and do not associate the experience of aversion and the negative feelings with other parts of their life, just with breastfeeding. Others have already been diagnosed with postnatal depression, but it is clear that the medication and treatment is not helping with their symptoms of aversion when the infant is latched, so they have gone back to the doctor. When breastfeeding mothers go to the doctor or paediatrician to disclose that they are having negative feelings when breastfeeding, they are sharing an important bit of information that can be used in a process of differential diagnosis. If aversion is a sign of struggling due to being triggered when breastfeeding as survivor of previous sexual abuse, or a sign of post-traumatic stress from an awful birth, or a sign that they have very painful feeds, these are all important. Aversion is an indicator for healthcare professionals that can help them arrive at a more accurate diagnosis than just labelling it 'postnatal depression'. The Catch-22 is that for doctors to be able to consider aversion as a medical sign, with specific symptoms, there needs to be clear, evidence-based information supporting the hypothesis. But there is little data, even fewer academic studies and no clinical studies, and subsequently there are no standardised assessments or screening tools, and no standard of care or treatment. They simply do not exist. Consequently, there isn't an acknowledgment of the phenomenon of aversion in the medical community, and it is not considered as part of the assessment process in lactation and health. In many ways this is unsurprising, because we know that there is a lack of good quality maternal breastfeeding and health assessment in general, as many health practitioners have little knowledge of or training in lactation.*

Until the case is made that aversion is important in the assessment and treatment of a mother and nursling dyad (pair), there is little justification to conduct medical studies on human participants, and it will be difficult to secure funding for the clinical data to be collected and an evidence-based approach to be worked out. The problem, like aversion itself, is cyclical. When you are in a situation where there is no 'disease' and no 'test', what is the next step? This book is an attempt to take the next step. I cannot deduce that aversion exists, because I don't have proof for it, least of all medical proof. I cannot necessarily infer that aversion exists, because there are not enough direct reasons to infer it from specific research that has been conducted on mothers who struggle with it. But I can abductively come to the conclusion that aversion exists, because there are enough pieces of observational information. This abductive approach begins with the mother's experience,

---

* Zakarija-Grković, I., Cattaneo, A., Bettinelli, M. E., Pilato, C., Vassallo, C., Borg Buontempo, M., Gray, H., Meynell, C., Wise, P., Harutyunyan, S., Rosin, S., Hemmelmayr, A., Šniukaitė-Adner, D., Arendt, M., & Gupta, A. (2020b). Are our babies off to a healthy start? The state of implementation of the Global strategy for infant and young child feeding in Europe. *International Breastfeeding Journal*, 15(1), 51. doi. org/10.1186/s13006-020-00282-z

the self-reported 'symptoms' of aversion we see everyday in the aversion community, and I have offered the most likely explanation for them, often starting with the simplest explanation. For example, if mother has a history of sexual abuse or baby is feeding with a restrictive tie causing persistent pain, a clear argument can be made for why aversion may occur, as there is an associative cause that we could attribute to the mother's negative emotions when considering body contact and the specific act of breastfeeding.

Unpicking your aversion

Currently, mothers are trying to self-assess their aversion, to figure out if it is part of their depression if they have it, or whether it can be attributed to a traumatic birth, a kind of PTSD of sorts. When supporting mothers with aversion I try to consider all the options, and start with the most common reasons that can be easily addressed, such as hydration and nutrition, as can be seen in Figure 5. If mothers have started to hydrate and eat better and their aversion doesn't go away, then we explore current and historical events, and pain levels. The reason why I do this should now be clear, as we have looked at a range of risk factors and underlying causes – it is a question of figuring them out for each individual mother. Aversion itself isn't necessarily the problem: it can be an indicator of other problems, though what these are will vary. The process of unpicking aversion helps us understand it, and will help you to understand yourself. Sometimes you are looking for something that is not obvious, or that you do not want to or cannot see, so you can tackle this by *ruling things out.*

Taking magnesium supplements is also a popular starting point, but they probably will not help you if you have uncomfortable or painful feeds, which suggests that there is something going on in the baby's mouth that needs addressing. Painful nipples can have many causes, and you will likely need a trained infant feeding professional to work it out. Sadly, your local doctor, even a paediatrician, is unlikely to be an infant feeding expert. If you experience aversion early

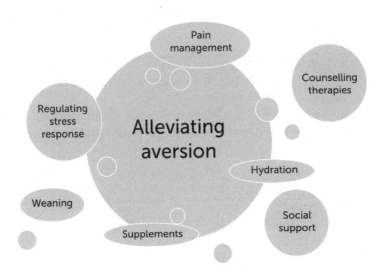

Figure 5: Options to Manage and Alleviate Aversion

on, when the baby is newborn, it is highly unlikely that it is a natural weaning trigger manifesting as maternal aggression, as we see in other parts of the mammalian world, because your baby needs milk to survive here. Weaning would make no biological or evolutionary sense. But if your nursling is older and your aversion is severe, it is likely the natural start of the weaning process: there may be an underlying biological change that we don't yet know about, but weaning is what your body is telling you to do, and you should consider this. Many mothers find it harder to manage the breastfeeding dynamic when aversion kicks in, as previously their nurslings would ask for milk, in their various and cute ways, and then get it. Learning to navigate a new dynamic can be hard, especially with toddlers who are unlikely to understand your pleas for empathy. In fact, before the age of two some argue nurslings cannot actually empathise, because those faculties have not developed in their brain. For this reason, older nurslings' behaviour can trigger aversion, particularly if you are in one of the at-risk groups. Somehow, we know when they are able to comprehend boundaries and adjust their behaviour. If you know what your triggers are, or you can look at what particular things stress you out, or what makes you upset, and why your mind turns on the negative story you replay in your head when breastfeeding, then you can recognise a pattern in what is happening with your aversion.

If during your self-assessment you cannot link aversion to ovulation or menstruation and the affects the related hormones can have, or your child isn't old enough for aversion to be a natural trigger to start the weaning process, you can think about the symptoms of aversion as an indicator that something else is going on. If you are in discomfort during a feed, or your nipples are very sensitive, might you be pregnant? If you are in pain, depending on the kind of pain, when it occurs and the severity, it may indicate a problem with the latch. Even pain when there is no visible injury or clear reason for it can be an indicator of other things and it is important to rule them out. And then there is the consideration of stress and how we deal with it: this can be the stress of experiencing pain when breastfeeding, or other forms of external life stressors, or even emotional stress. It is also important to remember that childhood trauma affects us in many ways, which come to the fore when you are feeling unhappy, trapped in a situation you cannot get out of, or stressed in life, and I believe aversion is one way in which this manifests.

If it is clear that your aversion isn't due to the risk factors, or a natural mechanism to start the process of weaning off the breast, then you can explore other areas of your personal, work or home life. As a new mother with a baby, questions I would ask include: are you managing all by yourself, or do you have anyone around? What did you think being a mother would be like, and what do you think babies should be like? Do you second-guess everything? How do you feel about mothering? Are these mothers in a constant state of mild stress, with elevated levels of cortisol that are having a negative effect on them over time? This last observation can apply to caring for older infants too. Do you struggle to bond with your older nursling when you are 'touched out' or stressed, and worry you may harm them if you withhold breastfeeding sessions or wean them off completely?

These questions open up the consideration of the indirect causes for aversion, such as your preconceptions of motherhood or your personal will and ability to cope with what breastfeeding can entail. Sometimes the causes are multiple and layered. It can be difficult at first to tease out what is causing aversion for you. But one thing we know for certain is that saying that aversion is a random occurrence, and that it is just something that 'happens', makes no sense, because too many of the symptoms can reasonably be attributed to biological causes or life events. So experiencing aversion is not just 'bad luck'. The good news is that this means that there is scope to alleviate aversion by changing how you think, what you do in your life, and even the way you eat, drink and sleep.

8

Alleviating Aversion

The basis of peer-to-peer mother support online, a sort of 21st century 'village', is that women can support each other through their joys and challenges in mothering, sharing experiences and invaluable knowledge. Online groups also offer solidarity in misery when aversion strikes. Our group 'Aversion Sucks' on Facebook even has a mentoring programme where mothers can get one-to-one support, and I personally go through the steps of navigating aversion as can be seen in Figure 6. Joining an aversion support group can help mothers to work through the process of self-assessment, which is specific to their situation, and help them change their circumstances. It is a safe outlet if they just need to vent to get through a breastfeeding session. An online aversion support group is an easy first step on the road to alleviating aversion, getting through aversion today, even getting rid of aversion entirely. Fighting the feelings of helplessness, gaining control of the situation and working towards breaking the cycle of negativity are all steps that are needed to help lessen aversion, and getting tips from peers can help you take those steps.

There are so many psychological, physiological and social factors that mothers are unaware of that might be factors in their aversion as seen in Figure 6. We have looked at them in detail, and I now suggest a number of steps to address aversion that are based on them, using an acronym I created BROMPHALICC.

Navigating Aversion

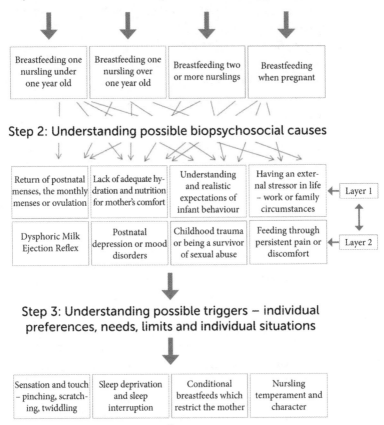

Step 1: What best descibes your breastfeeding situation?

| Breastfeeding one nursling under one year old | Breastfeeding one nursling over one year old | Breastfeeding two or more nurslings | Breastfeeding when pregnant |

Step 2: Understanding possible biopsychosocial causes

| Return of postnatal menses, the monthly menses or ovulation | Lack of adequate hydration and nutrition for mother's comfort | Understanding and realistic expectations of infant behaviour | Having an external stressor in life – work or family circumstances | ← Layer 1 |

| Dysphoric Milk Ejection Reflex | Postnatal depression or mood disorders | Childhood trauma or being a survivor of sexual abuse | Feeding through persistent pain or discomfort | ← Layer 2 |

Step 3: Understanding possible triggers – individual preferences, needs, limits and individual situations

| Sensation and touch – pinching, scratching, twiddling | Sleep deprivation and sleep interruption | Conditional breastfeeds which restrict the mother | Nursling temperament and character |

Step 4: Taking remedial steps to alleviate aversion

| Implementing the step-by-step BROMPHALICC method |

Figure 6: Navigating Aversion

This stands for:

- Breastfeeding aversion triggers
- Reactionary behaviours
- Ovulation and Menstruation tracking and management
- Prevention
- Hydration and nutrition
- Active distraction and redirection
- Lifestyle and sleep
- Interventional changes: mindfulness and minimalism
- Counselling
- Cessation of breastfeeding

Breastfeeding aversion triggers

The first thing I tend to ask when women reach out to me because they are having aversion is 'Do you want to be a mother right now?' And 'Are you happy, or is there something going on in your life?' I find that getting a broad picture of what is going on can put things into perspective. If the answer is 'no', or 'I'm not sure', then I know that aversion will likely have some roots in a psychological cause for this mother. There are so many things that we did before we became mothers that were exciting, fulfilling, and that gave us gratification and rewards, and we were able to pursue all of them if we wanted to. Living as a mother can be the total opposite of this for many women. Doing the dishes and cleaning up poop (we do a lot of this) is not as fulfilling or rewarding or complex as our lives before motherhood. University life, work life, and social life: all of these ensure, and even perpetuate and increase individualism and independence, not interdependence and personal restriction. The former are also reward-based. It would be naive and irresponsible to think that motherhood isn't significantly different, and that this does not affect the activity of breastfeeding for some women who find the transition difficult. So, the first step in tackling aversion is to go back to fundamentals in you and in the home to make sure we have them sorted out. Ask yourself, are you happy as a mother? Do you want to breastfeed, or do you *want* to want to breastfeed? Is there love, happiness and rhythm at home?

Or is there a daily drama, crying, and emotional hurricanes? If you are not happy, or you are, but not happy *being a mother*, and if there are difficulties at home, even though there may be steps you can take to alleviate aversion, it will be an uphill struggle because your relationship with your nursling is already strained. Trying to change the breastfeeding dynamic to get some freedom from your role and your burden may mean your nursling seeks more connection with you, which in turn will make you more frustrated, and your nursling's behaviour will start to reflect this, causing and perpetuating the vicious cycle of aversion.

Making changes without knowing your triggers

Without understanding the root cause of your aversion, you can compound your problems by trying to reduce or restrict feeds, and things could worsen. Imagine if you could change your mindset and alleviate your aversion? It would save you a lot of time and trouble. If you attempt to wean without working on a strong connection outside of breastfeeding, it can be really hard on both mother and nursling, and it often ends up not working the first time so you have to continue breastfeeding anyway. Then your aversion may become more severe as you feel increasingly trapped. Many women find that stopping breastfeeding to sleep because of aversion means they have to find another way to get their nursling to sleep, creating more stress and work for themselves. We may initially think that breastfeeding at night is causing aversion, only to realise once we night-wean that it is frustration with the multiple wake-ups, and the incessant and overwhelming night-time dependence on us that is causing the problem. Sometimes these frustrations reduce with night-weaning, but sometimes they do not.

What I am trying to get at is that there are always costs, and it is about weighing them up against what you would gain if you made changes. This is a hard calculation if you don't know what you are up against. Hopefully this book will have given you a broader understanding of the factors to consider when you make these decisions in your life. Often just having the words to understand why breastfeeding is so integral to our lives as mothers, with the concepts of nurture and skinship, can be helpful when you consider your aversion.

We have established that the symptoms of aversion could be an indication that there is something else going on, so how you get rid of aversion will depend on why you have it. To figure that out for yourself, I encourage you not to fixate on aversion itself, but to look beyond it and ask not only what your physical triggers are, but whether there is anything from your childhood and how your parents raised you that is still affecting you. How you were shaped and nurtured as a child directly affects how you parent, and not always in a good way.* Also, try to identify whether anything else has changed in your life lately that you think is unrelated, but could be causing you subconscious or low-level stress. Comments family members make about breastfeeding, or your nursling's behaviour changing to become more unpredictable as they grow through a developmental leap are common background stressors. Another thing to consider is any illness or teething, because this often means more requests to breastfeed, more time on you, and more chance of being 'touched out'. Not necessarily a good time to make changes to the breastfeeding relationship or start weaning.

Sometimes using psychoanalysis can help get to the root of your triggers, whether they be from childhood or current life events; you can use the principles of this therapy to begin to see how you interpret and respond to stressful situations. For example, if your nursling is crying and frustrated, and you cannot bear it so you try to stop them crying or tell them not to, it is likely that your mother or father did not allow you to cry or be frustrated. In a different way, other solution-focussed therapies, or cognitive behavioural therapies, can help re-route the way you think in order to change your behavioural response to a situation.** If you cannot afford counselling-

---

*   Perry, P. (2019). *The Book You Wish Your Parents Had Read (and Your Children Will Be Glad That You Did)*: (01 edition). Penguin Life.

** For self-help practical application see Ross M. D., C. A. (2009). *Trauma Model Therapy: A Treatment Approach for Trauma Dissociation and Complex Comorbidity*. Richardson, TX: Manitou Communications.

based treatment methods, and your local health provider cannot offer them, the first thing to do would be to talk to someone about your aversion, because secrecy never makes anything better. And in talking and having someone listen, we can often find our own triggers and causes of aversion.

Do not be ashamed of aversion: be frank, be honest, be raw. We have seen that emotions are not 'right' or 'wrong', but merely part of a breastfeeding mother's journey at different stages. If your situation is dire, or you need an intervention, or you worry about harming yourself or your child, then you really have to tell someone, ideally your doctor or another health professional. Otherwise, go to someone you trust first, show them this book, and use the words in this book to describe what is happening. Say 'I am struggling with breastfeeding triggering negative emotions, I have some unwanted intrusive thoughts, I want to push my child off me and run away'. Or 'I hate breastfeeding right now, but I don't want to stop', and 'I worry about the nights because I get angry and upset stuck in the room'. Or 'I feel like I am unable to regulate my emotions, I can't say no to breastfeeding because I don't know how to get them to sleep without breastfeeding'. Sharing this with trusted family members or friends, or even with other mothers who struggle with aversion in groups online, can really help. Like you, there are mothers across the world who have committed to breastfeeding – despite having aversion – in order to give their babies and children the milk and comfort they want and need. And there are mothers who needed to and have weaned because of aversion. If you are struggling with aversion to the point of wanting to night-wean or wean completely and your nursling is under a year old, then they will still need milk for survival and nutrition. It would be a good idea to seek professional advice from someone trained in lactation about how and when to abstain from feeding and how and when to supplement your nursling.

Struggling through aversion can be a soul-destroying experience; an existential crisis for a mother. As a group, mothers with aversion are hidden, so there are no regular meetings at which they can come together to share concerns and talk about what might help. Social media offers some safe and supportive environments where you can get the unconditional support of the people inside your phone, whatever time of day or night. There is always someone out there experiencing similar emotions to you, you just have to reach out to find them.

Triggers based on unrealistic expectations

Some breastfeeding support groups on Facebook have a mix of qualified infant feeding specialists called IBCLCs, breastfeeding counsellors and breastfeeding peer supporters who can relay accurate information about breastfeeding. If your heart and mind are appeased with information about biologically normal frequent feeds, or biologically normal frequent wakings at night, or perfectly normal disinterest in food when a child is teething or ill, then this may be enough to ease your frustration and lessen your aversion. Interacting with other mothers who understand the importance of breastfeeding and who are in similar situations does change things, because what other people say affects us greatly (this is in part why adverts are so powerful). I remember one mother who said she dealt with her night-time aversion by posting in a support group to ask how often other mothers' nurslings woke to breastfeed, and reading other mothers' comments that matched her nursling's behaviour. She then turned off parenting adverts on her social media accounts so that when she scrolled down her feed she wouldn't see images of babies sleeping or advice on how to get infants to sleep for 10–12 hours at night with a bottle of formula. If reassurance from others, alongside evidence-based information, changes your expectations and lessens your aversion, because it is happening to others and is more akin to your experience of breastfeeding, then this should be one of the first steps you take, as it costs nothing.

Reactionary behaviours

Prematurely de-latching can cause problems, and these problems change with age. Stopping feeds early if your baby is under a year old, and especially if they are under six months old, may compromise your nursling's nutritional intake, which they need to thrive. It may also compromise your supply, so it is a really good idea to get specialist breastfeeding support if your aversion is so severe that you are needing to do this frequently. If your nursling is over a year old and regularly takes food and water, reducing or restricting feeds may not put your nursling at risk, but that doesn't mean it will be easy. Working on de-latching with kindness, by giving nurslings an expectation that it may happen, will help. Although it can take time, working on other loving cues and creating another loving bonding attachment can shift the breastfeeding dynamic and really help break the vicious cycle of aversion:

> *Counting down from 60 seconds in my head helps me to keep her on longer, but by the time he was 13 months I could only bear ten seconds, and I would be saying it out loud by then, so we both knew what to expect. I found him to be less upset this way.* Rukaya, Dubai

It's much easier to work on your own reactionary behaviours before aversion gets really severe, because many mothers find they cannot respond calmly and lovingly at the same time as being 'touched out' and angry. De-latching in a calm and collected way means you are stopping any paroxysms of rage, and this can prevent the cycle continuing. When your nursling asks to feed, try saying 'Yes, but how about we do this first', instead of 'no', because this may be better received. Trying to stay away from places that make it easier to breastfeed, or just not sitting down when you know you can't bear to nurse can also prevent reactions. Structured deterrence and constantly distracting nurslings can be effective: if you are able to maintain conversation and interaction with them, do so very frequently. Talk about anything and everything you can think of, as a lot of the time if we are stressed we go quiet around our nurslings while our brains are tinkering away, and this means our social nervous system is offline. If we make ourselves have conversations with our nurslings, it turns that system back on, and also prevents us from placing ourselves in a situation in which we may react badly because we are triggered. If your communication is strong, then your relationship is strong, and if your relationship is strong, making changes or negotiating the breastfeeding relationship is easier for both of you.

'Love-bombing', and creating connection in another form, other than through breastfeeding, is possibly the cornerstone of navigating aversion with your nursling. It's terribly difficult to do when you are in the thick of it, because it's the antithesis of what you want: touch and closeness. Especially if it leads to requests for milk. It doesn't necessarily come easily, either, if you have deep triggers from your past or stress responses that you need to unlearn. It is particularly hard for some women when their nurslings react badly to being de-latched or being denied a breastfeed. Many of us have been parented in a way that makes it hard for us to listen to our nurslings' crying or emotional outbursts, but maintaining contact at that time can really help deepen the relationship. Their nurslings' reactionary behaviours to being denied the breast can make mothers very frustrated and upset too. But understanding that it is important to 'stay listening' to their upset in order to allow for connection afterward can help create another coping mechanism for mothers, instead of just breastfeeding:

> *I just couldn't bear all this screaming and crying. I kept telling him to stop but it would make it worse. It took me a while to just be able to sit and let him release all his anger at being taken off my breast, and to work through his pain, because I was so wrapped up in my own guilt.* Phoebe, Berlin

Using philosophies and teachings from organisations like Hand in Hand Parenting, and other attachment-focused approaches, can help you learn tried and trusted techniques that create a better understanding of your nursling and their needs. Changing the way you interact with your nursling, and changing how you de-latch, can reduce your aversion and change your nursling's responses and behaviour towards you, and subsequently around breastfeeding. Working on both their reactionary behaviours and your own can stop aversion becoming severe.

Ovulation and menstruation tracking

Aversion can strike once your postnatal menses have returned, and it's clear that hormonal and bodily changes have a role to play in this. Aversion for some women is a reaction to changes in their body. Not knowing this can mean your experience is unnecessarily worse. Some mothers feel more in control when they know their aversion is related to their menstrual cycle, and when to expect breastfeeding to get a bit more challenging. It also makes a big difference to know when it will come to an end! Tracking your cycle, noting the days you ovulate, and recording emotions and bodily sensitivity is essential to understanding your own menstrual pattern and working out whether your aversion is linked to these changes:

> *I fed my twins until they were two years old. When they were babies I never had aversion, it was only from when they were 18 months and onwards. I never knew about aversion, I just thought I was a really bad person for feeling like I did. It made me want to rip my babies from me and throw them across the room, the feelings were so intense! It was only when someone wrote on the aversion breastfeeding page on Facebook that it dawned on me what was happening. I recorded it and found it happened when I was ovulating; other times, it was fine, the feeding didn't bother me at all!* Henrietta, Lyon

If the spike of testosterone in your blood when you ovulate makes you feel particularly aggressive, it will be beneficial to keep track of your ovulation dates and make a plan to directly and proactively counter that testosterone peaking. As oxytocin is testosterone's direct antagonist, getting the 'love' hormone flowing in a positive way will do wonders. Just steer clear of conventional advice to do skin-to-skin breastfeeding, as this can exacerbate the situation! Bodily contact like short bursts of rough and tumble play, which doesn't result in requests for breastfeeding, will mean nurslings are engaged without being at the breast, and is known to build connection.* Loving touch from another adult that doesn't trigger you can also be effective, as it is known that hugs anywhere lasting from three to 20 seconds can reduce stress, help us release oxytocin and change a negative state.** If you aren't normally one to instigate touch, try to force yourself to. A hug from a person we love and trust will change our biological state instantly, and it is worth doing frequently when struggling with aversion.

When we consider oxytocin release related to our menses, the positive effects of the hormone are only responsible for lowering a woman's stress for part of her cycle. It is the social bonding of interacting with others, with self-nurturing and self-care, that stimulates the hormone progesterone, which can lower a woman's stress during the rest of her monthly cycle. These hormonal shifts need to be supported by the presence of other people, otherwise her own testosterone goes up and her oestrogen reduces and she feels stressed. This stress spills over to our nurslings, and can make breastfeeding less enjoyable if we get aversion.

If your menses are painful and difficult to manage, some naturopathic herbs and remedies have been shown to be effective,*** especially evening primrose oil.**** Working on making your period less of a physical and emotional disruption will help if you struggle with them monthly. Reducing stress triggers and the pressure on yourself can help you cope during this time; not planning to do too much on those days, and ensuring you allow time for rest and recuperation. We have

---

* Cohen Ph. D., L. J. (2012). *Playful Parenting* (Reprint edition). Ballantine Books Inc.
** Hugs help protect against stress, infection, say researchers. (n.d.). Retrieved 17 October 2019, from ScienceDaily website: https://www.sciencedaily.com/releases/2014/12/141217101316.htm
*** Mirabi, P., Alamolhoda, S. H., Esmaeilzadeh, S., & Mojab, F. (2014). Effect of Medicinal Herbs on Primary Dysmenorrhoea- a Systematic Review. *Iranian Journal of Pharmaceutical Research : IJPR*, *13*(3), 757–767.
****Mahboubi, M. (2019). Evening Primrose (Oenothera biennis) Oil in Management of Female Ailments. *Journal of Menopausal Medicine*, *25*(2), 74–82.

mostly moved away from periods being shameful, as women were made to believe in the past, and we have products to help us manage the bleeding and hygiene so that we can carry on as normal. However, we haven't yet managed to learn to listen to our bodies while we are menstruating, to allow our bodies to go through the process with ease. It can help to allow ourselves the time and space to bleed and comfortably, quickly and easily access bathrooms to clean ourselves. If you have heavy periods, not going out and about when you don't need to will make life easier for you, especially if you have a nursling. It is a matter of making adjustments during your menses to see if these have an effect and lessen your aversion.

Prevention

Sometimes there are very definite things that can help with aversion and may prevent it. For example, tandem-feeding mothers who begin feeding their nurslings singly may no longer experience it at all. At other times mothers can work on accepting their body's reaction to breastfeeding and say 'this is okay' without being overwhelmed by the emotions, and without being plagued by guilt and shame. Accepting aversion is certainly one way of alleviating its grip on you and your nursling, but that doesn't mean it is easy to do, as this mother says:

> I tri-fed, which means I pumped, breastfed and formula fed. I had no sleep, I mean none, I was in so much pain, I used to walk around with no bra on at home. I was desperate, and alone, I hated breastfeeding then. To me anger was a reasonable reaction. But I couldn't own my own anger, because I was being crushed by a fantasy. I had to be happy, I had to enjoy breastfeeding, I had to enjoy being a mother. It took me months to let go and start to accept it for what it was: hard work. Elena, London

Managing your own expectations and anger is important so that you don't have your nursling's mirror neurons firing and mimicking what you do, compromising the social nervous system and your home environment. But in order to self-manage, many mothers need support from another adult, and distance from their nurslings, to regroup. And not just occasionally, but in a consistent and structured way so that it can be nourishing and restorative. Otherwise, negative social emotions spread around the house, and it can quickly become unmanageable. Another reason for having another adult or person around for support and for company is not for you, but for your nursling. One of the hardest things about aversion is that hugs and loving gestures often lead to nurslings asking for milk.

When I tried to reduce feeds I thought I could swap them for hugs, how wrong I was! It seemed every time we were hugging there would be this awful tug of war to get to my breasts between me and her, and it always ended in tears, for both of us. Aversion is so cruel, I can't breastfeed her and now I can't even hug her! Emily, San Francisco

The habitual patterns of nurture and skinship, and the strong attachment oxytocin has helped to foster, are very important in the breastfeeding relationship. Making adjustments so that you respond to your nurslings in a way you can manage while not triggering aversion is the goal of any physical intervention to help with aversion, but the better goal to aim for is not to get aversion in the first place. In order that changing the breastfeeding relationship is easy on everyone, preventing aversion is key, no matter how old your nursling is. Introducing 'waiting hands',* breastfeeding manners and alternative sleep cues can help to prevent aversion, although these strategies may take some time to work effectively. Humans are creatures of habit, so start to implement habits that can create mini pockets of freedom for you: a few minutes here and there is enough to start with.

---

* 'Introducing Waiting Hands' found (n.d.). Retrieved 23 October 2019, from Playing with Chanel website: www.playingwithchanel.com/home/2018/6/30/waiting-hands

In general, whether mothers are considering weaning or not, I usually always suggest introducing other sleep cues, including having a lovey or a cuddly toy, and a particular song or word you use *every single time* they are going to sleep. The idea is that they associate these things with sleep, so you have a cue you can use that isn't breastfeeding. When the time comes to wean nurslings from breastfeeding to sleep you then have other options that you have already introduced.[*] Alongside this, working on having trusted people become part of the caring environment during the day and night is important to allow for a safety net if aversion strikes or becomes severe, or just so that you can take an actual break or have a good block of sleep. Introducing sleep cues and another trusted caregiver takes effort and time, especially since nurslings' development and patterns are changing and often unpredictable. Don't expect anything to happen quickly, but when it does, you will reap the rewards.

Working on your own ability to relax, and increase your oxytocin is another key prevention strategy. As oxytocin is a very powerful hormone that can override stressful states, but also trigger them, it needs to be manipulated in order for it to work for you – you need to bring it under your control, and this can also take time.[**] Accessing positive oxytocin associations in yourself can be tricky when you are trapped in the vicious cycle of aversion. Consider what is associated with breastfeeding, and thus oxytocin, when you have aversion: negative emotions, tension and stress. Start by looking at whether you are positively or negatively pairing oxytocin, and find what feels good for you to help change it. This might mean increasing body contact that you find pleasant, and happily consent to, that brings smiles and laughter. Being able to do this is often the result of other things that you can work on, such as how you feel about your life, or being able to reduce other stresses at home. Before being able to work

---

[*] Hookway, Lyndsey. (2018). *Holistic Sleep Coaching – Gentle Alternatives To Sleep Training: For health & childcare professionals*: Praeclarus Press.

[**] Reversing oxytocin pairing in D-MER can take time, and multiple treatments including counselling and manipulating the mother's environment, for those with severe aversion the same could be true.

on positive contact you may have to make concerted efforts to change your home environment and your mood, perhaps lifting it by using music, aromatherapy, yoga, or love-bombing before, after or during any physical contact with your nurslings in order to positively pair oxytocin. Again, this is not a quick fix, but rather a commitment to changing the home dynamic and your mindset in order to alleviate aversion. Remember that you are in charge of your emotions, and you can take steps to look at what makes you happy: a chat with an old friend, taking a minute for yourself, getting active, smelling certain scents or eating chocolate. Do them all, as often as you can. Anything you can manage to change your mood and increase your oxytocin. If you are in a slump, get up and jump up and down: putting on your favourite song will get you moving and change your physiology. Persistently working on your mood can prevent aversion, and prevent it from worsening if it already exists.

It is hard to make a shift, and if you are persistently feeling hopeless and as though you can't work on these things, this may be an indication that you need more intensive support. Seek advice from a lactation or medical specialist, being clear and open about having aversion and any other information you think is relevant from your past to help them properly and accurately assess the situation. It may be that you have an underlying clinical condition that you have not thought to rule out, or you have brushed off. Depression, anxiety and mood disorders are common medical conditions that are co-occurring, especially in the postnatal period. Seeking out screening and assessment for postnatal depression can be a starting point. Some mothers are reluctant to consider this because they do not want to take medication when breastfeeding, as there is a common myth that breastfeeding is not compatible with taking certain drugs. This is simply not true.[*] Many antidepressants, and other drugs used to treat various medical conditions, are completely safe for breastfeeding mothers.

One of mothers' main fears about aversion is that their

---

[*]   Jones, W. (2013). *Breastfeeding and Medication* (1st edition). London: Routledge.

negative response to breastfeeding will turn into a negative response to their nursling. So it is always worth implementing changes to prevent aversion from getting worse. Prevention is almost always better than treatment or cure, but sometimes this is not possible. There are many things you can do straight away if aversion strikes, which address different parts of the biopsychosocial phenomenon. Starting with what you eat and drink.

Hydration and nutrition

If you think that what you eat and drink cannot affect you in health-changing, mood-changing ways, think again! I've stopped being surprised about the role of food and drink in health, because over the years I've read thousands of clinical trial protocols as part of my role as vice-chair of a research ethics committee at the Health Research Authority. When investigating a new drug, study participants are routinely not allowed to ingest certain things, including caffeine, poppy seeds and grapefruit, and all the meals on a clinical trials unit are strictly monitored. Any non-adherence means that participants are excluded from the trial. Why, I hear you ask? Well, because food and drink affect your body at a pharmacological level. This micro level is where drug interactions in your body are measured, and the science of how it works is called pharmacokinetics.

Many foods and naturally occurring substances can affect homeostatic balance in our bodies, to the extent that they can skew clinical trial study findings. In fact, many clinical trials monitor and manage the food intake of the clinical trial participants to record any changes in the body and to see the specific effects on the study drug. Food is not only responsible for homeostatic and pharmacological changes, but also changes to our mood: even our decisions are linked to what we consume. This is in part, because of our microbiome. The 21st century has brought an eruption of research into the real 'brain' of the body. Our gut appears to be the mastermind in control of our bodies. Groundbreaking research has shown how our gut health may affect whether we are depressed or if we get fat.[*]

Furthermore, your environment and circumstances affect what you choose to eat. This is certainly the case for the sleep-deprived mother. Research shows that if you are sleep-deprived you will opt for fattier and higher sugar-content breakfast foods in the morning, even when ordinarily you wouldn't start your day with those options.[**],[***] As sleep-deprived mothers we may continue to make these decisions for weeks, months or years if we are breastfeeding day and night. It's no surprise that mothers describe themselves as living on coffee and cake. This combination may 'get us through the day', but what are the long-term effects, and how are these foods affecting how we feel and behave? How are they affecting breastfeeding? Eating poorly does not do much for your mental health, and we know that weight and mood can affect our hormones. And as hormones play a role in aversion, it is wise to work on eating a well-balanced diet if you are prone to choose high sugar and fatty foods due to sleep deprivation.

There are certain essential nutrients that we all need in order to survive and thrive. Zinc and magnesium, for example, are considered key elements in the human body, as more than 300 enzymes require zinc and magnesium to perform their activities. Etebary and colleagues found that zinc and magnesium are essential both in neurotransmitter production and in the regulation of their release. As zinc and magnesium can have an antidepressant effect through neurotransmitters like serotonin, a severe deficiency in zinc is thought to be a risk factor for depression and other neurodegenerative disorders.[****] Morns, a public health nutritionist, and the

---

[*] Enders, G., (2014) *Gut: The inside story of our body's most under-rated organ*: New revised and expanded edition: Scribe Publishers.

[**] Brondel, L., Romer, M. A., Nougues, P. M., Touyarou, P., & Davenne, D. (2010). Acute partial sleep deprivation increases food intake in healthy men. *The American Journal of Clinical Nutrition, 91*(6), 1550–1559.

[***] Rihm, J. S., Menz, M. M., Schultz, H., Bruder, L., Schilbach, L., Schmid, S. M., & Peters, J. (2018). Sleep deprivation selectively up-regulates an amygdala-hypothalamic circuit involved in food reward. *BioRxiv*, 245845.

[****] Etebary, S., Nikseresht, S., Sadeghipour, H. R., & Zarrindast, M. R. (2010). Postpartum depression and role of serum trace elements. *Irani-*

founder of the first nursing aversion support group on social media, suggests that naturopathic support including the use of supplements like magnesium may help aversion in mothers who are tandem feeding.* Taking certain supplements does help some mothers, but we have to remember that the placebo effect of supplements and pharmaceuticals can be as high as 30–40 percent. Furthermore, if your aversion is due to persistent pain, discomfort while breastfeeding through pregnancy or previous sexual abuse, taking supplements may not help you, because they cannot change the underlying cause of your aversion. If you choose to try supplements, it is always best to see a trained specialist in naturopathic approaches or a conventional doctor who is knowledgeable about evidence-based treatments that are not pharmacological. However, there is nothing stopping you from changing your diet to include vitamin- and nutrient-rich foods every day, or taking a daily over-the-counter supplement and seeing if this lessens your aversion. There is a lot of research that indicates that mineral supplements like magnesium and zinc are effective in the treatment of many medical conditions, and there is strong anecdotal evidence it helps some mothers in the aversion community. It is only a matter of time before we have peer-reviewed evidence to back this up.

Next, make sure you are well hydrated and drinking enough to maintain adequate fluid levels in your body. We lose fluid in many ways, through sweating, urinating and even though our faeces, which are one-third water. As breastfeeding mothers who make milk, eat more, and poop more, we lose more water. So breastfeeding mothers are at risk of mild dehydration.**,*** Some women find that their aversion lessens or even disappears when they hydrate frequently. It is known

an *Journal of Psychiatry*, 5(2), 40–46.

* Morns, Melissa, & Steel, A. (2018). Naturopathic support for nursing aversion associated with tandem breastfeeding. *Australian Journal of Herbal and Naturopathic Medicine*, 30(2), 74.

** Zorc, J. J., Alpern, E. R., Brown, L. W., Loomes, K. M., Marino, B. S., & Mollen, C. J. (2012). *Schwartz's Clinical Handbook of Pediatrics* (5 edition). Lippincott Williams & Wilkins. 4th Edition,p296.

*** Ibid p297

that oxytocin aids the let-down of the milk, and has also been found to make mothers feel thirsty,* which makes sense given that breastfeeding works on a supply and demand cycle. If you don't notice your thirst, or it lessens as your baby grows, it is important to stay well hydrated when you are struggling with aversion:

> *I used to get aversion really badly at night until someone in the group suggested hydrating. Usually, I can't drink at night, because I'm stuck in one position and I can't reach the water bottle. So I found one which is spill proof, so I can keep it next to me all night, and that has a camel-neck lever so I can even drink it lying down.* Nadia, Sicily

Even though we know that being mildly dehydrated does not affect your milk *supply*, that doesn't necessarily mean it won't affect *you* and your emotional resilience in mothering. And if you are a busy mother who struggles to finish a cup of tea without it going cold, by the time evening comes, not only might you not have drunk the daily recommended amount of fluid, but you might also have had four slices of cake or two packs of biscuits! So whenever you breastfeed, hydrate. Ideally drink something without sugar and caffeine in it at least once a day. No one is suggesting you have to give up the tea, or the cola, completely!

Active distraction, boundary-setting and redirection

Boundary-setting is often suggested for mothers of older nurslings, but what isn't often discussed is that setting boundaries takes time, consistency and usually only works if it is done with kindness. For this reason, it's ideal to start boundary setting early on, because it takes a lot of effort to

---

*   Information, N. C. for B., Pike, U. S. N. L. of M. 8600 R., MD, B., & Usa, 20894. (2009). *The physiological basis of breastfeeding.* Infant and Young Child Feeding: Model Chapter for Textbooks for Medical Students and Allied Health Professionals. The Physiological Basis for Breastfeeding, session 2.

focus on it later when you are struggling with aversion. Nonetheless, starting at any time can really help to bring the equilibrium back into the breastfeeding relationship:

> *I started doing waiting hands with my toddler, which helped me loads when I just need a moment to gather myself. I want him to get the idea of waiting for a moment for me to fetch something or if I needed to prepare to breastfeed. I also only breastfed on a particular sofa in the living room, or chair in the bedroom . . . so he started to understand there were some restrictions.* Emma, Brighton

The first thing that is really challenging when boundary-setting is giving love to, or consoling your nursling, without them asking for the breast, particularly if you have triggers for aversion around the way you are being touched. Doing your utmost to prevent access to your skin can help: one mother said she would wear a polo neck even in the height of summer just so her breasts were not visible. Always hug when fully clothed on top if touch triggers you. Holding and kissing while walking up and down can calm nurslings – this sometimes works and means they do not ask to feed because you are not sitting down. Motion and contact together are very powerful for calming nurslings and getting them to stop crying. If the contact still ends up in requests for the breast, there is no harm in using a home pushchair to create motion and calmness without contact, and without breastfeeding. If your nursling is old enough to be eating and drinking, stocking up on their favourite food is often helpful when you know aversion will strike, or if you are trying to reduce and restrict breastfeeding sessions. Whether it is fruit, raisins, or baby 'biscuits' that don't contain sugar, many nurslings are happy to sit with you and eat instead of breastfeeding (at least until they finish them!). Giving these snacks may be the lesser of two evils if you are experiencing aversion, particularly if it is severe.

The second thing that is challenging is getting your nursling to sleep. Although some may consider it a faux pas, using a 'home' pushchair or a sling to get your nursling to sleep can work, and avoids the breastfeeding-to-sleep-marathons that can become volatile due to aversion. Temporarily delaying bedtime until they are completely exhausted and fall asleep in minutes can also help to re-regulate a nursling's sleep and mean they do not breastfeed for two or three hours at bedtime. Aversion is side-stepped. These measures should be used while addressing sleep hygiene at home and working on loving de-latching. Basically, use whatever tools you can in order to achieve your goal of calming, connecting and responding to your nursling until you can get on top of what is causing your aversion and sort it out:

> *Touch was affecting me in a bad way, but I couldn't stop breastfeeding, so I wore multiple layers all the time so grabbing at my breasts was almost impossible and skin contact very minimal. I would wait until she was so exhausted to allow her to feed from me, that way after a few minutes she would knock out and I would barely have to deal with aversion.*
> Alice, Calais

Distraction

When aversion strikes you may find you reach for your phone, knowing that you cannot survive breastfeeding without scrolling or playing Tetris. Many women will instinctively distract themselves in order to be able to cope with and temper their negative emotions. This is *cognitive distraction:* we actively divert our mental attention. Cognitive distraction is the go-to tool for mothers with aversion, because it's free, has instant effects – you forget about your intrusive thoughts and negative emotions – and it works. The science behind it is that your brain cannot focus on more than one cognitive activity at a time. So if you are looking at posts on Facebook, watching your favourite series, or playing one-handed Tetris, your brain doesn't have the cognitive ability to dwell on the emotions that are at risk of spilling over when you are breastfeeding. Studies indicate that even a two-minute distraction is sufficient to break the urge to ruminate. So each time aversion strikes, use distraction techniques or force yourself to concentrate on something else until the urge passes. Of course, the problem with this is that when you stop distracting yourself, as you invariably do, the aversion resurfaces.

Aversion that doesn't go away is also attritional, which means it can get worse over time, and for some women who hit their breaking point, distraction will no longer work. Additionally, night-time exposure to blue light from screens can suppress the production of melatonin and affect the quality of your sleep. Distracting yourself for a two-hour breastfeeding-to-sleep-marathon with your phone, and then during every feed at night, will invariably affect your sleep hygiene and therefore sleep itself, so it is wise to be cautious. Sleep hygiene refers to habits and behaviours around sleep that are conducive to getting us to feel sleepy and have good quality sleep: they should be consistent, calming, confident, and help you feel connected. Listening to something with headphones that engages you in a calm way, or using a stress ball or fidget device in your hand may prevent the negative effects on sleep of using a phone.

Along with cognitive distraction, *physical distraction* can help mothers get through a feed. Using this 'gate control' method can be instantly effective and has been used to manage pain by selective stimulation for many decades – because non-painful sensations can be used to override painful ones. You may find, as many mothers do, that you dig your nails into your thighs, or cup and squeeze your breast firmly, while your nursling is latched, just to get rid of the irritating sensations of suckling or the uncomfortable contact on your nipple. This kind of physical distraction works and is really effective because it creates a stronger physical sensation elsewhere in the body that overrides the irritation of suckling, meaning you focus on the greater discomfort or sensation. It also creates a state of control, because *you* are creating the sensations, *you* are controlling how much pressure to apply and where. You create a stronger sensation in an area that is not overly sensitive, so it can be tolerated more easily, depending on how long a feed can last, and how severe your aversion is. If aversion is severe, some mothers will self-harm out of desperation, just to be able to cope with a nursling latched and suckling. If you pinch yourself or dig your nails into your skin to the point of drawing blood, it would be wise to consider finding other distraction techniques to get through a feed, or consider reducing feeds in a consistent and safe way. Remember, aversion can be your body's way of telling you to make a change.

Using the tool of distraction applies to your nursling too: if your nursling is older than a year, you can start implementing it. Many mothers spend a lot of time alone with their nurslings, without others around to help meet the considerable need for interaction and attention that many nurslings have. With breastfeeding so interlinked with nurture and skinship, we may find that breastfeeding on demand continues to be a frequent activity as our nurslings get older, despite their need for the actual milk being less. Making plans to be out and about, where there are other adults and children to distract from requests to breastfeed, can help you get through a day. Distracting by offering healthy snacks, water or food before feeding can sometimes work too, but if aversion has become severe, more intensive distraction activities should be employed that make you both feel a bit calmer and more connected, in order to prevent your nursling asking to feed and the vicious cycle kicking in.

Lifestyle and sleep

We know from research into cancer and heart disease that lifestyle categorically affects health. What you do, what you eat, whether you exercise and even how you think over the course of your life has a direct impact on your health. Although breastfeeding itself has been found to have protective effects against breast and ovarian cancer, and protects against maternal mental illness,[*] we cannot escape the pressures of modernity and modern lifestyles do affect us and put us at

---

[*] World Breastfeeding Trends initiative, 2016. Retrieved from ukbreast-feedingtrends.files.wordpress.com/2017/03/wbti-uk-report-2016-part-1-14-2-17.pdf

risk of poorer health. I listened to a BBC Radio 4 programme called *Why Can't Our Children Talk* recently, about how the pervasive use of screens, and even central heating, is being blamed for speech problems in children that can affect them their whole adult life – from their mental health to their earning potential.[*] Another insight was that in the future we may have fewer skilled surgeons as manual dexterity and coordination declines due to an over-reliance on screens. One expert claimed that trainee surgeons won't be able to sew or cut with accuracy, a key part of this highly skilled profession.[**]

A critical area in which lifestyle affects us is sleep and sleep quality, and aversion can be worse when we are sleep deprived. Have you heard of the term 'hangry'? It is a portmanteau word made up of 'hunger' and 'angry' and refers to the state some people get into when they are hungry, which doesn't dissipate until after they have eaten. I want to propose the term 'slanger', for sleep-deprivation and anger. It is unclear to me why there hasn't been much research in this area, because it seems like a common phenomenon. Perhaps it is because it predominantly affects women when they become mothers, which is not a major area of interest in our rather patriarchal, male-led society. A recent critically acclaimed book by Professor Matthew Walker called *Why We Sleep*, citing all the latest research on how sleep affects humans, makes little reference to mothers, let alone breastfeeding mothers, who are perhaps one of the most sleep-deprived cohorts in the entire population! It is an exceptional book, but one that left me rather annoyed.

If you are a mother, you are most likely sleep deprived, and if you get aversion when breastfeeding, it's not unreasonable to think there is a link. How dependent you are on sleep may mean you are in the group of mothers who really cannot cope with little sleep and broken nights. In addition to being angrier when sleep deprived, if you routinely use your phone

[*] BBC Radio 4—Why Can't Our Children Talk? (n.d.). Retrieved 18 October 2019, from BBC website: www.bbc.co.uk/programmes/m0002b-mv

[**] Coughlan, S. (2018, October 30). Surgery students 'losing dexterity to sew'. *BBC News*. Retrieved from www.bbc.com/news/education-46019429

to distract yourself at night, and if you get aversion particularly at night, both the nocturnal adrenalin and the blue light from the screen will inhibit getting to sleep and staying asleep. If your parasympathetic nervous system is online and your social nervous system is online you and your body are in a conducive state to enjoy deep, restful sleep – even if it is interrupted by breastfeeding occasionally. If you experience aversion, however, a stress response is triggered when breastfeeding, and your sympathetic nervous system is activated. Moreover, if you have negative association with oxytocin, the let-down when you are breastfeeding will further inhibit your ability to relax as the stress response is triggered. It is also well known that the big players in social media have intentionally sought to create artificial dopamine hits that are designed to keep us coming back for more. With constant exposure to screens, and staying up, we have to be careful not to dysregulate our carefully balanced sleep systems that rely on melatonin.

Melatonin has a relaxing, hypnotic effect, and tampering with its production and release can interfere with our ability to get to sleep and stay asleep. It is known that breastfeeding exclusively is associated with longer sleep at night in nurslings, because breastmilk at night contains higher levels of melatonin. Melatonin is secreted by adults but not nurslings, and as we know it is key for sleep, it is thought that it passes into nurslings through the milk.[*] Whereas melatonin has been shown to govern the sleep/wake cycle, it is serotonin which is the key hormone in wakefulness, triggering sleep and the deep REM part of sleep. Serotonin levels in particular parts of the brain also affect our mood, which is why low serotonin levels (as seen in people with depression and anxiety) lead to sleep problems. Exercising can help produce and regulate your body's serotonin levels. Yet, as mothers we often become more sedentary. Our bodies may have changed in pregnancy, and our eating habits change too, particularly when lacking sleep. Coupled with the lack of movement breastfeeding

---

[*]   Cohen Engler, A., Hadash, A., Shehadeh, N., & Pillar, G. (2012). Breastfeeding may improve nocturnal sleep and reduce infantile colic: Potential role of breast milk melatonin. *European Journal of Pediatrics*, *171*(4), 729–732.

can entail, we may put on weight without noticing. Without structured routines of 9–5 work and ongoing social plans, and with the new routines of caring for our nurslings that take up all our time, the limited amount of time we have for ourselves may mean that exercise disappears from our lives. This can compound our problems, particularly if we are sleep deprived, because the serotonin produced during exercise helps make melatonin, which cues which your body and mind to get ready for sleep.

If the idea of going to the gym makes you cringe, or a yoga class is impossible due to childcare, and frankly you never feel like exercising because you are too tired, then you are in luck. We live in a marketing age where the first principle of selling is to 'give for free', and so we have great resources on YouTube, where expert trainers and instructors provide exercise videos that you can do in the comfort of your own home, without the need for the faff of a gym. In fact, some research shows that just five to seven minutes a day is enough to see beneficial effects, and doing five to seven minutes a day is certainly enough to build on. It's not getting through the short videos that is the difficulty, but starting them, and with free 'get fit challenges' online that step is almost eliminated. The idea is that you can start to change your lifestyle habits by laying foundations that you can build on to help your mood and your sleep.

We know that good sleep habits are important for good quality sleep, so consider your sleep hygiene. This means all the things you do to maintain a good sleeping environment and get ready for bed. When asked 'Why do we need to sleep?', William Dement, who founded Stanford University's Sleep Centre and who has researched sleep for the last 50 years, replied 'As far as I know, the only reason we need to sleep that is really, really solid, is because we get sleepy.'* So the getting sleepy bit is really key, not only for us, but for our nurslings. Unfortunately, 21st-century life has absolutely everything on offer to prevent that from happening. Lights, internet, home

---

* The Secrets of Sleep (2010, May 1). Retrieved 22 October 2019, from Magazine website: www.nationalgeographic.com/magazine/2010/05/sleep

delivery. Our fast-paced, constantly interactive life affects our mental state and our sleep. The modern-day phenomenon of stress has crept into all our lives, whether we like it or not. And stress is really the antithesis of sleep. So, in addition to doing a teeny bit of exercise each day, start implementing good sleep hygiene. Put yourself and your family first over an imaginary person on a TV show, or even a real person on social media. That can all wait.

Your evening should start with around two hours of dimmer lighting and decreased stimulation, which will allow you and your nursling to calm down and be ready to get *sleepy.* This is a big commitment, and can mean changing the way the family lives, by shifting when you do activities, when you eat and when you relax; consistency is key. The early evenings should be consistent, calming, connecting and ideally co-parented, so everyone winds down to get *sleepy.*

If you are overtired and running on adrenaline, having repeated releases of cortisol throughout the day, the longer you delay getting ready for sleep the less likely it is you will be able sleep. Neither you nor your child will be able to 'get sleepy', and all the breastfeeding in the world won't help. Well, maybe three hours of it will, but by then you are a wreck, full of rage, and even more tired and frustrated than before you started the bedtime routine.

According to Lyndsey Hookway, a holistic sleep specialist, to bring balance to things at home you can make bedtime later in this situation, but just temporarily. This is called bedtime fading, and it can correct the faulty sleep hygiene that has crept into the family home. The main aim is to prevent the rapid sleep onset when infants and toddlers fall asleep within 10–15 minutes, as this means they are massively overtired. This is the same for you: when you are overtired and feeling stressed, sleep interference will be rife and will affect your breastfeeding ability. This, and any anxiety in the environment of sleep, will make your sleep and their sleep much worse. As co-parenting was found to be an independent variable to the quality of

---

*   Hookway, Lyndsey. (2018). *Holistic Sleep Coaching - Gentle Alternatives To Sleep Training: For health & childcare professionals*: Praeclarus Press.

infant sleep, managing the family home can be key to reducing nurslings' dependence on you at night, and consequently help you manage your aversion.* Sometimes, when infants wake at night, it has nothing to do with them, but with the atmosphere they are in. Teamwork, rather than bickering with harsh words, and rash dialogue, is sometimes what you need for nurslings to sleep well. If you want to lessen night feeds with the aim of improving your nursling's sleep, it is important to change the way you do things during the day and at bedtime first, and monitor what happens. Just stopping breastfeeding at night doesn't always improve your nursling's sleep, so you will be just as sleep deprived. Addressing sleep hygiene can mean ruling out as much as you can in your home environment that is affecting you all. Focusing on sleep hygiene can mean a big commitment to change, but it will be worth it. Like anything, it will take time to learn and form new, better habits, but at least this way you are able to reconnect with what you really need, what your body is telling you when you have aversion and emotions that might be linked to *slanger*.

So lifestyle and sleep can affect your breastfeeding, and your happiness while breastfeeding. If you have little to no spare time, and many external commitments, it can be difficult to sit and breastfeed responsively without feeling the tug of needing to 'do something else' and subsequently getting restless and agitated. Honouring your sensitive self and living a slower, more intentional life is hard for some mothers, especially when our 'old' habits from life before children creep in. But if you are struggling with life as a mother, and your body is trying to 'say no' (as I believe it is when you get aversion), it might be wise to listen to that inner voice. It's okay to say no to that invitation if you know it's going to drain you. You don't have to have your kids signed up for every sport and extracurricular activity that comes around. You are not obliged to help run everything you're involved in. When we are stretched too thin, it takes a toll on our already sensitive nervous systems as mothers who are primary caregivers and always 'on call'.

When there are no blank spaces in the calendar, there is

* Ibid

no room for lounging around, catching up on basics that need to be done like the washing up, or just recharging. The idea here is to make choices that fit into your new life as a mother, with its new responsibilities and restrictions. Having a child, or children, will inevitably bring a great deal of restriction, particularly in the beginning, especially if you are not surrounded by family or structured support so you can have regular breaks. Shifting your lifestyle to have minimal commitments and pressure, if you can, in any area of your daily life, will help create more space. This will in turn create more time and allow you to breathe a little when breastfeeding.

Interventions: mindfulness and minimalism

Mindfulness

Dr Jill Bolte Taylor, a neuroanatomist, who hypothesised about the '90-second rule', states in her book that our neuropathways actually only fire for 90 seconds, which means your actual neurobiological response to something is only 90 seconds long.[*] Anything more is just your story, replaying in your head. The response you have after that minute and a half is you choosing to carry on with that response. If we consider a mild trigger in aversion, say a sensation like pinching, or the thought of having to wash the dishes, the negative knee-jerk reaction on a neurobiological level according to this theory should only last 90 seconds. It is the tendency for some of us mothers to ruminate that makes aversion, in that specific instance, worse. Using mindfulness can be a powerful way to downregulate your negative response by stopping the replay of your 'story' in your head. Learning how to handle your strong emotions using mindfulness techniques, and deep breathing, can help you ride the worst waves of negative emotions aversion can bring. On many occasions I used Buteyko breathing to get a handle on aversion, as it is one of the easiest and quickest ways to get control over our autonomic nervous system and induce

---

[*]   Bolte Taylor, J. (2009). *My Stroke of Insight*. London: A Brain Scientist's Personal Journey', Hodder Paperbacks.

a parasympathetic state of relaxation.* Many mothers I support use the app Headspace to start with if they have not had any experience with breathing and mindfulness practice, and it can certainly help lessen aversion if it is not yet severe. (It can take time to master these techniques, and it may not help if aversion strikes out of the blue.) Nevertheless, like any of these interventions, it is so important to start to implement them as soon as possible, so you can get better at managing aversion in the long run, especially if you have aversion repeatedly or continually and do not want to wean or your nursling is very resistant to weaning.

Curbing your response is so much easier when someone else is around, like a partner or family member who you can be yourself around, and who understands what aversion is. I have often thought that mothers shouldn't be left alone to deal with such a big burden if they are struggling with breastfeeding, especially aversion, because some of them simply cannot manage it alone. The stress of experiencing negative emotions can invariably build if you do not have a support network, but it can become intolerable if you are literally alone at home all day, and all night. And although the role oxytocin can play in aversion may mean a stress response is continually triggered alongside breastfeeding, research has found that practising mindfulness can give you the tools to reduce the effects of stress, and your stress responses. Moberg and Kendall-Tackett, when writing about the negative feelings women with D-MER have, believe mindfulness can help downregulate an overactive stress response, especially when combined with a kind of counselling called cognitive behavioural therapy (CBT).** They state it is effective in the treatment of post-traumatic stress disorder, but maintain that this technique can apply to any negative stress responses as they have similar pathways in our body through the autonomic nervous system.

*   Russo, M. A., Santarelli, D. M., & O'Rourke, D. (2017). The physiological effects of slow breathing in the healthy human. *Breathe*, 13(4), 298–309.
** Uvnäs-Moberg, K., & Kendall-Tackett, K. (2018). The Mystery of D-MER: What Can Hormonal Research Tell Us About Dysphoric Milk-Ejection Reflex? *Clinical Lactation*, 9(1), 23–29.

When the parasympathetic nervous system is activated, we are rested and can be relaxed. Our adrenaline and cortisol is controlled and not spiralling, our saliva production is normal and even increases, our pupils are normal, our heart rate is resting and our breathing rate is normal. Oxytocin is not inhibited. When the sympathetic nervous system is activated (as I believe it is when aversion strikes) the opposite things happen: saliva production slows, we get a dry mouth that often occurs when stressed or sleep deprived,* and our pupils become dilated as stress hormones are released. Our heart rate then increases and so does our breathing rate. We start to take shorter, shallower breaths, often without noticing. In this state oxytocin is restricted and cannot function the way we need it to as mothers with dependant nurslings.

So how do we reactivate oxytocin, achieve homeostatic calm and re-regulate our emotions? The answer is by bringing our consciousness to the tension in our body, and by breathing deeply with long exhalations to slow our heart rate down. Then we can use our breath to engage mindfulness to stop the negative chatter in our minds. Again this kind of practice takes time, but it is worth implementing to tackle negative emotions. If you are new to it, or you are stuck in your negative loop, you can begin by focussing on relaxing music, or using your voice to change your mood and put your social nervous system back online. Don't think, just put on a song you like and make yourself sing. The muscles used in speech, the pharynx and the larynx are the same as those used in singing, and can shift our interactions with others and ourselves, which is why talking therapies can be so effective as treatment, and why they help relax us. Being alone as a breastfeeding mother can mean you don't have anyone to talk to, and can make things worse because variations in pitch and tone from others' voices mean we have to listen with focus, and this in turn will engage the social nervous system again. Talking, or singing, requires

---

*   Villa, A., Connell, C. L., & Abati, S. (2014a). Diagnosis and management of xerostomia and hyposalivation. *Therapeutics and Clinical Risk Management, 11*, 45–51.

coordinated breath and relaxation, which will in turn become relaxing. And using our voice is not only a tool to relax ourselves as mothers, singing has also been used for centuries to help calm and soothe babies and children. Sing to your nursling if you are inclined, and if you can't, just talk to them. Talking and chatting gives nurslings a flow of safe cues, their response will be engaged and bring smiles, which will further perpetuate positive emotional contagions at home. The idea is to nurture mother and nursling, with them responding to each other in a fluid and dynamic way, and having a positive impact on each other. This is one reason why research shows that breastfeeding protects against maternal mental illness *when it is going well.* When breastfeeding isn't going well, it doesn't have this effect. Aversion is one example of when it's not going well, and can be a sign of other difficulties that are affecting breastfeeding.

While seemingly simple solutions like breathing and mindfulness can and do work if applied consistently, there are other factors that affect aversion and they too need to be addressed if this approach is to work. We know that expectations from society and those we put on ourselves can prevent us from slowing down when we need to. We need time to adjust, to recover, to embrace the changes of matrescence we have gone through and fully embrace what is normal in motherhood. A lot of research shows that adverts - which we are constantly exposed to – can affect our emotions, as these are a key component in buying decisions.* Companies spend millions of pounds each year on making marketing effective, so it is not a stretch to think that they may play a role in triggering a mother's negative emotions when breastfeeding, especially if those adverts show non-realistic idealised images of mothering. Mothers are constantly shown what they 'should' be experiencing, and their reality does not match

---

* LaBarge, M. C., & Godek, J. (n.d.). (2006) *Mothers, Food, Love and Career-The Four Major Guilt Groups? The Differential Effects of Guilt Appeals.* 2. Advances in Consumer Research Volume 33, eds. Connie Pechmann and Linda Price, Duluth, MN : Association for Consumer Research, Pages: 511-511.

it. The products they are bombarded with claim to make life easier, better and happier. Often this means that our house starts to become full of useless clutter. Clutter that are often reminders of what we tried with our nurslings that didn't work like moses baskets and expensive white cots.

Minimalism

The more stuff you have, the more time you have to spend cleaning and sorting it. The more things you do, like activities and social meets, the more time and energy it takes from your day. This is where the concept of minimalism comes in. An online survey of women who breastfed showed that the amount of time they spent every day breastfeeding varied from four hours to over seven hours a day.[*] The time varied depending on the age of the infant and what was going on in the life of the infant, such as developmental leaps and teething, illness, and other socio-demographic circumstances of the mother: if she was a stay-at-home mother, or at work, and if she had other children or needs. Whether it is four hours or seven hours, breastfeeding is time-consuming. How much time you spend depends on where you are in your breastfeeding journey, and the severity of aversion varies according to how difficult you find it to spend time breastfeeding. Adopting a minimalist mindset can help. Minimalism is about not only objects, but also things that do not serve you in life, whether it is friends, habits, objects, foods or activities. Even 'parenting' theories. If they do not suit you or your family, let them go. If you simplify your world, you allow time for breastfeeding and the nurture and skinship that come with it. You can respond to your nursling regardless of how often they ask to suckle and concentrate on changing the dynamic if you need to.

> *It's like I woke up and found that the person I once was had gone and a mother had replaced her. And what made it harder was that everything around me at home and everyone outside reminded me of the 'her' who had gone. I wish I had*

---

[*] Survey on the online resource site www.breastfeedingaversion.com, conducted from unique site visitors between 2018-2019.

taken steps in my life to make space for that mother before she arrived. Gabriella, Galway

Opting for a minimalist approach to life can therefore help with stress, even just in regard to objects and 'stuff': if you minimise your surroundings, you are not looking at chaos or clutter, and not constantly being reminded of all the things you need to do. There are many studies showing how having less stuff means having less stress, which is better for you, and even your nurslings. One study even suggests that having fewer toys makes children more imaginative and is better for their cognitive development, having a more positive impact at home than the densely crowded playrooms most children have.[*] Creating a positive home environment that accommodates your personal sensitivities is important for self-managing aversion, because nurslings can pick up on your tension or tension in the home. Minimalism allows you to clear out all the distractions, and everything that steals your energy, so you can start to know yourself, and your nurslings better. Find what feels good for you, and start with the little things. Maybe change the lighting, from neon bright lights to daylight bulbs and even red night lights. Essential oil diffusers with lavender oil, calming music: introduce anything that may help you make positive associations with breastfeeding and help you get through a feed. Knowing yourself is crucial to coping, as it will help you monitor your triggers and also curb your responses. Knowing when to say no, knowing what depletes you and what helps re-energise you, and how you centre yourself can be life-changing. It can be a lot of work to change, and it depends how much you want it, but acknowledging that some things in your life may need to change in order for your aversion to lessen can help if the cause of your aversion isn't deeper and more traumatic. In this case you may need some form of counselling to help.

---

[*] Dauch, C., Imwalle, M., Ocasio, B., & Metz, A. E. (2018). The influence of the number of toys in the environment on toddlers' play. *Infant Behavior and Development, 50*, 78–87.

Counselling and other therapies

We can try to tell ourselves that no feelings are wrong feelings, and that 'this time when I breastfeed it will be different', but when we end up getting aversion or acting on the negative feelings the emotional loop of guilt continues even when we are not breastfeeding. If the aversion cycle continues, many women feel that it seems to take over their daily lives. They begin to think about hating breastfeeding even when they aren't doing it, and they start to *dread* the next feed.* It's just how all of our brains work: we tend to focus on the negative as humans, so one tip is to record small wins. Write it down if you breastfeed your nursling without aversion, so you can focus on the positive and retrain your brain to remember it. In life, as in aversion, nothing happens all of the time so exceptions are what you look for. Keeping a record of the 'good stuff' is often part of therapy, and there are many types of counselling that can be useful to get to the root of your struggles: whether it be your relationship with your parents, events that happened to you as a child or past and recent trauma. Even though I argue that for some women the symptoms of aversion are a physiological response to a lack of control and compromised autonomy around her breasts and body, or a stress response running concurrently to breastfeeding, aversion is a biopsychosocial phenomenon – so counselling can help change the way you think and thus your physiological response to a situation. For example, sexual abuse and its interplay with anxiety, depression and sleep problems is a key factor in those women's experience of aversion. And although women in this group are more likely to report a desire to breastfeed than formula feed, they may have hypersensitive feelings to it or find themselves triggered and may need help to manage this.** It would be difficult to do this alone without some sort of objective insight to identify what is going on when triggered, and how to prevent escalation. In these mothers, counselling-based therapies could be a way to address aversion.

---

*   Even the next pumping session.
**   And not only because of deep ingrained hypersensitivity to stress-ors, but also society at large plays a role because breasts have been over-sexualised.

Talking therapies like solution-focused approaches and methods like technical rewind techniques that combat stress and anxiety* can work for many reasons, because they help us understand the way we think. If you have found through reading this book that your aversion has links to birth trauma, rebirthing may help you to sustain your breastfeeding journey and tackle the root of aversion. Other therapies like cognitive behavioural therapy work on changing how we act by focussing on what we think about certain parts of our life. Sometimes, we are the obstacle that sits in the way of change, but we don't know it. Finding a solution is not possible because we will not budge on a certain point – often for good reason. Counselling therapies work by helping us move past being 'stuck' in ourselves, being stuck in our past, even being stuck in a present problem. If you are really brave, psychoanalysis can get to very deep-rooted beliefs you hold and the reactions you have to them when they present themselves in a different life situation. Some mothers have certainly found this helpful when struggling with breastfeeding challenges.

Other mothers have tried the emotional freedom technique (EFT) or 'tapping', which is a quick, easy, non-invasive treatment that can help to regulate and release emotions in the moment. Tapping can be self-administered so you can try it today to help you with aversion by finding easy to follow tutorials online. While it does not get to the root causes like other counselling-based therapies, it can help manage and channel the waves of emotion that aversion brings.

Counselling for pain management

Despite it being a difficult experience, being in hospital as a child taught me a great many things, one of which relates to when I used to say I was in pain as a minor and wasn't believed. This made me realise that pain is really your own body talking to you – only you and no one else. It is a language the body uses to communicate to us, but we are not able to

---

* Griffin, J., & Tyrrell, I. (2006). *How to Master Anxiety: All You Need to Know to Overcome Stress, Panic Attacks, Trauma, Phobias, Obsessions and More*. Chalvington, East Sussex: HG Publishing.

pass that knowledge on so effectively.* The likelihood of getting aversion may increase depending on how sensitive it feels for you when you are breastfeeding or being touched in general (ie, time of the month). Although nipple pain is common in the first eight weeks postnatally, for mothers who struggle with persistent discomfort or pain after this period, whether due to menstrual cycle sensitivities, an undiagnosed reason, or falling pregnant, part of what can enable them to cope with pain is their commitment to breastfeeding, and acceptance of the pain. This is important if aversion strikes, because emotions like anger and sadness from pain can also cause pain in some medical conditions as they promote inflammation,** and we know these emotions mean more cortisol is released. Ongoing or 'chronic' pain has significant personal and social impact, and we know that distress and pain are associated with depression, anxiety and a decreased quality of life. Psychological therapeutic treatments like CBT have been widely used in other chronic pain-related conditions and have shown effectiveness, but without a clinical trial we won't be able to say for certain if they will help with breastfeeding pain or aversion. A popular CBT method called acceptance and commitment therapy (ACT) would be an ideal tool for mothers in the situation of aversion when they cannot wean, as ACT invites people to open up to unpleasant feelings, and learn not to overreact to them, and not avoid situations where they are invoked. Its therapeutic effect is a positive spiral in which feeling better leads to a better understanding of the truth of the situation faced by the individual, and a way to manage persistent pain – although clinical data is needed for its efficacy in breastfeeding mothers struggling with aversion. Another promising area is a self-management intervention for breast and nipple pain that has recently been developed and

---

* Variations of physical touch and sensory stimulation, and issues around sensitive areas particularly the nipples is one clear reason some breastfeeding mothers do not want to be touched in those areas.

** Graham-Engeland, J.E., Song, S., Mathur, A., Wagstaff, D.A., Klein, L.C., Whetzel, C., & Ayoub, W.T. (2018). Emotional State Can Affect Inflammatory Responses to Pain Among Rheumatoid Arthritis Patients: Preliminary Findings. *Psychological Reports*, 33294118796655.

shows efficacy for mothers to use their knowledge, beliefs and social support to reach their breastfeeding goals.[*]

Therapies for trauma

For women whose aversion is linked to trauma, a therapy called eye movement desensitization and reprocessing (EMDR) might help. EMDR has been found in clinical trials to be effective in the treatment of emotional trauma and adverse life experiences. There have also been numerous studies showing it to have a more rapid effect than cognitive behavioural therapy, with decreases in negative emotions, somatic complaints, recall and intensity of memories.[**] Experiential contributors and clinical manifestations of EMDR work by changing a perceived threat into something you can manage in a physical as well as psychological way. Given that aversion has both psychological and physiological symptoms, which can be seen from observation and mothers' own reports to stem from adverse life experiences, EDMR therapy may well help with alleviating or lessening aversion. Until we have published research showing clearly that one type of counselling treatment works for mothers who struggle with aversion, we have to rely on inferring that it may help by looking at the other conditions they are used for. Anecdotally at least, mothers I have supported have found counselling and other therapies useful. When they do not work, and the other approaches we have considered do not work either, I believe the only solution is weaning.

Cessation of breastfeeding

We now know that for some mothers, breastfeeding, the tool they have to create a bond, to nurture, to quiet and console,

[*]   Lucas, R., Bernier, K., Perry, M., Evans, H., Ramesh, D., Young, E., …
      Starkweather, A. (2019). Promoting self-management of breast and
      nipple pain in breastfeeding women: Protocol of a pilot randomized
      controlled trial. *Research in Nursing & Health*, *42*(3), 176–188.
[**] Shapiro, F. (2014). The Role of Eye Movement Desensitization and Re-
      processing (EMDR) Therapy in Medicine: Addressing the Psychologi-
      cal and Physical Symptoms Stemming from Adverse Life Experiences.
      The Permanente Journal, *18*(1), 71–77.

to have intimacy and skinship, is – with aversion – the very thing that is sabotaging the mother-nursing relationship. Breastfeeding as the cure and the cause is a terrible situation for a mother. Severe aversion is a Catch-22: there is no possible solution, because of the way breastfeeding relates to mothering, skinship and nurture. Instead of a win-win scenario – we know that breastfeeding benefits and protects nurslings, as well as protecting mothers against breast and ovarian cancer – it turns into a zero-sum game. One person's gain means another's loss, making the net change in benefit zero. We are used to thinking of breastfeeding in terms of a specific mechanical activity: the production and transference of milk that sustains life and aids development. But we do not make decisions in relation to this production and transference of human milk: breastfeeding has multifactorial importance and how we feed our nurslings is complex. This includes not only emotions, but that these mothers are identified by breastfeeding, that these mothers *rely* on breastfeeding, and that their nurslings do too. These are all major obstacles to weaning.

Weaning is always an option when experiencing aversion, but despite what healthcare professionals and most of society tend to suggest, it is neither the first resort, nor is it without consequence. People should not advise weaning under the following naive assumptions:

1. It is *easy* to do.
2. It is *better* for mothers and/or nurslings to stop breastfeeding.
3. Infants *will* 'take a bottle' (many refuse, and repeatedly).
4. That toddlers *should* 'take a bottle' (follow-on milk is not needed and toddlers can be introduced to cups).
5. It doesn't bring up other problems (ie, how does one settle one's child to sleep if they have been breastfed to sleep prior to weaning off the breast? How does one comfort an infant when they are hurt or scared in the interim when weaning? How does one create another 'bonding' practice when they have previously had the

closeness and familiarity of breastfeeding?*').

6. It doesn't have risk of low mood, or weaning depression for the mother – because ending breastfeeding completely – even if it isn't abrupt can cause depressive symptoms and sadness.

7. It is fine to switch to pumping. While some mothers can breastfeed easily and have no problems with supply, some of these same mothers find it difficult to express or haven't the resilience to pump daily. Some even get aversion when they pump, so may have to source human milk elsewhere or use formula, both of which have risks attached.

Considering all of the above seriously means weaning is often neither appropriate nor straightforward. Even without the difficulties of aversion, women have stated they find it unhelpful when people, especially healthcare practitioners, suggest they stop breastfeeding.**,*** Weaning itself can also be a tiresome and emotionally draining process, which can take weeks, months, or even years of gentle trying. Mothers can have a strong attachment to breastfeeding too, which will be there despite aversion, because of oxytocin and the bonds it has created tying you to the activity. The bond, and oxytocin, keep you doing it, despite the pain, and negative feelings – it is not a matter of 'just' stopping. The role that oxytocin plays is critical in aversion: it simultaneously creates the calm and closeness, making us attached to our nurslings through breastfeeding, as well as our primal instinct to protect. It seems the latter feelings are still being evoked even if we have a stress response to what's going on, but in a misplaced way. There is

---

* On this it is just as naive to think these don't affect the mother or the family balance and home life, these factors can make daily struggles worse.

** Attard Montalto, S., Borg, H., Buttigieg-Said, M., & Clemmer, E. J. (2010). Incorrect advice: The most significant negative determinant on breast feeding in Malta. *Midwifery*, 26(1), e6–e13.

*** Hauck, Y. L., Blixt, I., Hildingsson, I., Gallagher, L., Rubertsson, C., Thomson, B., & Lewis, L. (2016). Australian, Irish and Swedish women's perceptions of what assisted them to breastfeed for six months: Exploratory design using critical incident technique. *BMC Public Health, 16.*

a difference between the way females and males respond to these kinds of situations. Part of our fight or flight response as females is to befriend, nurture and be the caregiver – even in difficult or painful situations – because of the amount of oxytocin that is produced. We problem-solve through the emotional abilities we have, and the attachment we have due to oxytocin. For males this stress response will be directly in the area of fight or flight; they will be quicker to anger and quicker to action, which is perhaps why many male partners of mothers struggling with aversion will suggest weaning and even become impatient if they do not. Levels of oxytocin in any situation an individual finds stressful will also be high, and if this is a prolonged or repeated event, it may have an addictive element. Oxytocin also crystallises emotional memories and solidifies relationships, which is why the bond between mothers and nurslings is so strong, and perhaps another reason why breastfeeding is in some ways addictive for both parties. This explains why we can't let go of it as breastfeeding mothers, even if we find it difficult, even if we experience persistent pain, even if we experience aversion.

Typically, you would think that if something or someone was hurting you or making you uncomfortable, you would want to step away, but mothers who go through aversion seemingly become more and more engrossed in the breastfeeding relationship. The worse the aversion gets, the more stressful it gets, the more they are binding to breastfeeding because of the role of oxytocin. Although they want to wean on one level, they are also developing a fear of the future without breastfeeding or worrying about the unknown harm they may do to their nurslings by weaning before they are ready to. Stopping breastfeeding can be a very real fear, so there is a slippery slope and a snowball effect. Every time we think of leaving or stopping, we remember how important breastfeeding is and go back to our deeply ingrained habitual behaviours and thoughts. We have a habit that has been attached to a very strong bond created by oxytocin – whether positively or negatively associated, it is still a bond. Habits are very difficult to change. Not only are you more attached to the breastfeeding relationship, your maternal instinct is operating on overdrive. You literally prioritise your nursling due to breastfeeding and the associated biological pathways that reinforce it: the nursling becomes the most important object in your perceived world.* This understanding of aversion and the role oxytocin plays goes some way to explaining why mothers can't just remove themselves from tricky situations and 'get out', or 'just stop' breastfeeding. Their persistence may come, in part, from this hormonal pathway, regardless of whether aversion is acute or chronic. The development of this attachment through breastfeeding, and its habitual practice, means that when you think about leaving your nursling and stopping breastfeeding, you have an immediate direct stress and fear response that cripples you and holds you in the situation. In the right situation, and with breastfeeding going well, oxytocin plays a critical role in the development of a strong relationship with your nursling, but in difficult situations I believe it plays a critical role in the development of aversion. So you are not a monster, you don't just have psychological 'issues': you could actually have a biological mechanism that explains why you are experiencing aversion and are struggling to stop breastfeeding. My best suggestion is to deal with this situation as you would deal with any other habitual 'addictive' practice that was causing some level of distress or harm, using the general approach of addiction theory. You have to understand habitual practice, understand the biology that lies behind it, identify your own personal triggers, address them and consider the costs of continuing or stopping. When you are physically and emotionally suffering because of using substances as an addict, it is time to make a change. Similarly, if you are physically and emotionally suffering because of breastfeeding, and you

---

*   Being independent outside the context of the breastfeeding relationship becomes difficult because the relationship is extremely co-dependent. The mother, as a result of the oxytocin production in a stressful situation, can create social avoidance and social anxiety situations. They don't leave their homes and their quality of life diminishes over time, as the antisocial component, when it is attached to stress memories, perpetuates a complete state of helplessness. So the oxytocin production makes breastfeeding more habitual, more 'addictive' if you like.

have exhausted other options, I would consider it the same. Sometimes making changes and setting limits and boundaries when breastfeeding works, but if your nursling is not amenable to this, or your aversion is too severe or has gone on for too long, the only answer left may be to wean.

We have seen that weaning is not an easy choice, and it comes with its own risks and costs to you and your nursling. Expectations play a large role in how smoothly weaning off the breast goes and we often have some (very reasonable) expectations around weaning as mothers, given that we have spent hundreds, sometimes thousands of hours breastfeeding over many years. We perhaps expect our nurslings will stop sooner, or we do not expect them to go absolutely crazy when we stop them from breastfeeding at any one time. We could expect it would be easier to say no, expect them to understand our pain, expect they would behave rationally, or simply just expect it to be easier to do. Many mothers feel these difficulties force them into an 'all-or-nothing' situation: the inconsistency of not being able to offer the breast due to aversion and premature de-latching means the nursling's reactions worsen because they are not getting clear messages about what you want and what they can do. Many mothers don't want to stop breastfeeding altogether, but just to breastfeed less or not at night. Yet, for some nurslings breastfeeding is definitely an all-or-nothing thing. It's either accessible all the time and on demand or there is a massive meltdown. For mothers of these nurslings trying to reduce or shorten feeds actually makes the whole situation worse, even though neither the nursling nor the mother wants to stop breastfeeding altogether. But if the vicious cycle of aversion repeats, it is no good for anyone. De-latching will happen. If you can't manage gentle de-latching, distracting your nursling, lowering your voice, having calm connection, listening to their outpourings and all the rest, then it may be time to consider stopping breastfeeding. You can start anytime with a conversation, a plan to reduce feeds, to have someone else do bedtime, and the introduction of other dependency cues. Crying in arms, and staying present when saying no, will ensure nurslings are not left feeling abandoned when they experience a change in the relationship. To wean takes commitment and consistency, particularly if your nursling is very attached to breastfeeding. To ensure being able to follow through on your decision, I have tried to write about the cessation of weaning in a frank way, being honest about the pros and cons. This is because we need to be sure we truly want to wean, and we need to give ourselves permission to do it.

Aversion and its perpetuation can sometimes be more about you: your actions, your responses, your connection with your nursling and how able you are to manage your emotions. Can you *respond* not react, can you take heed before you speak, can you not take their behaviour personally? Are you able to reframe their determination to feed regardless of your needs as a phase, or even as them testing the boundaries of the world? Can you acknowledge and engage their suffering, or is your suffering too overwhelming, your story too full of hurt? If you cannot, you may be in an 'intolerable situation', where nothing you seem to do or say helps you out of it. Weaning will be the answer to your aversion, but the dynamic in your relationship with your nursling will still need some work. These intolerable situations can and do exist in life, and motherhood is one area where they are likely to be present because of conflicting needs and the strain that mothering can put on almost all aspects of life.

9

Intolerable Situations

Before aversion, my breastfeeding goal was to feed my two daughters until they decided they no longer want my milk. Aversion is the intruder! The saboteur! Aversion is the unexpected circumstance that compromises me from achieving my breastfeeding goals. Giving in to these sometimes overwhelming symptoms without weighing up my options first, may be just as harmful. For me it would mean not being true to myself. Bekka, Germany

Not being able to nurture through breastfeeding, and having skinship compromised by aversion, makes decision-making as a mother very difficult. It is natural for mothers to want to rid themselves of aversion when it strikes. But sometimes, when mothers turn to breastfeeding peers in real or online groups and disclose aversion, they are met with statements like 'this too shall pass', which makes me despair. A mother with severe aversion is *in crisis*. I see a lot of posts in parenting groups that say the worst thing to tell a toddler in a tantrum is to 'calm down', yet we do much worse to grown adult women who are in dire straits as mothers, admitting their feelings, thoughts and aversion experiences in groups online. 'This is wrong', 'How can you say that about breastfeeding your child?', 'Get some help', 'Delete this post', 'Call child safeguarding' are typical responses I have seen. How will this help someone in an emotional crisis?

I think the posters who comment as I mentioned above

could do to reflect on the famous quote '*Homo sum, humani nihil a me alienum puto*' ('I am human, and nothing human is alien to me') by Publius Terentius Afer, a Roman playwright during the Roman Republic. Human nature, and human needs almost always take priority over the moral imperative if a difficult situation arises. His point is that you should never really rule out thinking or doing something that you currently judge as being wrong, because the human condition dictates that you *could* think or behave in a different way if circumstances dictated. To those mothers who are adamant they would never raise their hand to strike their child, or who say they would never, ever resort to cry it out, I would say: *I wouldn't be so sure of yourself.* You have no way of knowing how you would react given enough pressure or restriction, if you had had a different childhood or traumatic experiences, or you were simply so sleep-deprived you were beside yourself with despair. Unless you have lived through these things, like that person reaching out in desperation, you will not know and cannot say that you would 'never do such and such'. And if you cannot empathise or understand a mother's reaction in such difficult circumstances *for her*, it only tells me you have been fortunate enough *not* to be in the same circumstances, under the same conditions. Whether you *ought* to behave differently or 'better' as a desperate mother in any given scenario or situation is, frankly, a discussion for the moral philosophising ivory tower academics who have neither the time, interest, nor theoretical and methodological capacity to apply real-life occurrences to their logical and rational thinking processes. You 'ought' to be a better mother, you 'ought' to control your negative emotions, you 'ought' to breastfeed through it, you 'ought' not to night-wean if they need it, you 'ought' to try harder, you 'ought' to change your self-care and not sleep train . . . It doesn't matter what you 'ought' to do! As mothers we do what we have to do to survive, not just physically, but psychologically and emotionally – and that will almost always mean that someone suffers, either ourselves or our children or our partners, or all of them. We will fail, if somewhat temporarily, because no one can win all the time with an uncertain set of circumstances, competing and conflicting needs, with unknown variables, unpredictable changes and limited energy. You just can't. Unless you are a Kardashian, or a Royal and you can buy the help you need. You can buy the options you don't have, you can buy freedom, you can buy sleep, you can buy time for your mental or physical health, and you can buy happiness in motherhood. They can, you can't. You are now a mother, you have to carry on now, it's all on you, and when you experience aversion but you cannot 'just stop' breastfeeding, this is abundantly clear. Some mothers have burdens that they find too heavy to bear. Aversion can be a manifestation of this. This sense of breastfeeding as a burden becomes ever more apparent as there are more and more restrictions on health budgets, with key services being cut, including maternal health and breastfeeding support services. That is why this book is about understanding aversion yourself, and navigating through it yourself in the first instance. Figuring out if it is something you can change, or reaching out if you need to get professional help.

The principal rule of thumb through this book was one of 'parsimony' – when applied to a situation, it is the rule of finding the easiest, simplest explanation and solution. I have tried to apply this approach to understanding different parts of the phenomenon of aversion, and helping you understand it. When you *feel* like you are stuck like a prisoner, you will become unhappy and agitated, especially if you feel you cannot do anything about it and you have no control over it in the short or long term. Or, if breastfeeding is painful, you will have an aversion toward it, and if you persist while being in pain, you will likely become agitated and angry while doing it, perhaps even feel a little crazy. These things are not 'bad' or insignificant. If you are just utterly disappointed with your life as a mother, your expectations were crushed when you started to live the reality of motherhood in the 21st century and you lament the loss of your previous life of freedom and independence, then consider that this experience has a role in your aversion. It takes quite some time to even recognise yourself and your body as a mother – when you look in the mirror and what you see is not who you were in years gone by. Taking these realisations a step further, I would ask yourself honestly, are you even happy? Do you want to be a mother? Are there things in life that really bother you, but when you think about them, they are lifestyle or mothering goals that you have inherited because of the age we were born into, with its societal pressures? Is your aversion actually a normal reaction that anyone in your situation would have, or is something from your present or past interfering with your happiness and ability to mother right now? Sometimes, expensive psychoanalysis isn't needed to tease these things out; sometimes three months of CBT is unnecessary. If you can write down what is happening to you, it would be a start in addressing your aversion, your personal triggers, your personal causes. Sometimes, the plain and simple truths are easy to understand – though I am not saying that they are easy to change.

Being honest with yourself

Only once you have acknowledged some personal truths and they are out in the open can you know what you should do about them. What are your truths, if you were really honest with yourself? One 'truth' could be that you just do not want to be there, at home. You don't want to spend time with your nurslings alone in the house; you would rather be at work, or with friends. Or a 'truth' could simply be that you just don't want to breastfeed. You may *want* to want to breastfeed, but deep down you hate it, and aversion is that spilling over. Another 'truth' could be that you are unfulfilled, bored, or even that you feel you do not love your child as you are meant to. Or perhaps you feel breastfeeding and mothering is just not worth it, as you get no reward, or there is no reciprocity? To find out a truthful answer to this, you could ask yourself: 'If I was getting paid £5,000 a week to do what I am doing right now, would I do a better job? Would I be less resentful? Would I feel as 'touched out', or experience negative emotions when breastfeeding?' Some high-end nannies make over £100,000 a year to care for young children day and night. Thinking about it honestly, would you feel the money would make it worth it? Thought experiments like this are interesting for a number of reasons. They turn your assumptions and conclusions about what you think – and who you think you are – inside out, they offer an alternative way of looking at a situation and they often allow you to come up with a deeper understanding of yourself, different options and creative answers to problems. When experiencing negative emotions, there may be many layers of self-deceit to uncover.

Aversion can be very complex, as can be seen in Figure 6 on page 179, and most women cannot just take a pill to sort it out. Although magnesium supplements do work, they only work for some mothers, and this is for a reason. If you have specific triggers from past trauma, magnesium will do nothing to abate them and your aversion will remain. The environment around you is also very important in influencing whether aversion manifests, as we have seen. Having company and a helping hand or being alone while mothering during the day/night can mean the difference between being happy and coping with breastfeeding, or unhappy and struggling with it. How you have been brought up will affect you too – if there was any failure of attachment with your parents, or if you experienced childhood trauma or abuse, your ability and resilience in being able to cope with stress will be impacted. And then there are so many points in the journey of becoming a mother that can be stressful. When we look back at how our social nervous system works, we can see that your unconscious responses to a situation, unbeknown to you, are making it worse. The way you react when they cry, *how* you de-latch them with a smile or a scowl, and whether you are able to smile, laugh and play during the day with your nurslings will have a direct impact on your breastfeeding relationship – and on your nurslings' behaviour with you. It is the difference between preventing aversion or making it worse.

Your previous losses and painful experiences in life can distort your perception of the world and also your interactions with your nursling – without you being able to stop it – because you do not know how else to be. Perhaps no one has showed you, perhaps you haven't seen mothering first hand, or perhaps you are just overwhelmed with the transition to motherhood and the loss of your old self. This loss includes major parts of life: your independence, for example, both physically and often financially, and also your body as you knew and (wished you had) loved it. The Egyptian novelist Naguib Mahfouz wrote that nothing records the effects of a sad life as graphically as the human body, and nowhere is this more vivid than in the scars mothers have. The changes in their body happen alongside a reduced ability to live how they used to. When becoming mothers women may lose their health, their beauty, their wealth, their friendships. They lose their time, their personal space, often their intimacy or relationship with their partner. This amounts to a loss of 'self'. Things haven't just changed in your body and in your life; there has been a deep loss. You have lost someone very dear to you, you have lost a person you once were, and right now it seems there is nothing you can do to get her back. Things are hard, you are stuck, you are angry and resentful deep down inside, but you do not know it, as many of us do not know that *anger's real name is grief*. Aversion on this deeper level is a manifestation of grieving the loss of self, and the loss of the dreamy world of expectation that is replaced by grim reality. The negative emotions of anger and agitation sit well within the understanding that there are different stages of grief, including denial, depression and acceptance. Denial about what has happened to us as mothers, that some of us are not depressed but *motherhood sure is depressing* when it is difficult, and the bittersweet taste of acceptance of your lot when nothing you do seems to work. Having persistent aversion, and not being able to wean for whatever reason, is the epitome of being stuck between a rock and a hard place. Shivam Rachana, an international author[*] and birthing trainer, teaches how pre- and postnatal experiences, birth trauma and obstetric violence can affect mothers and babies post-delivery.

---

[*]   Rachana, S. (2000). *Lotus Birth*. Victoria, Australia: Greenwood Press.

Postnatal depression is a healthy response to this experience, which requires appropriate attention and healing, not just treating of the symptoms.

An appropriate response to an intolerable situation

Is aversion just an appropriate response to an intolerable situation for a mother? In many ways, I believe aversion is an entirely normal response to a situation with a particular set of conflicting demands and difficulties. Women who experience persistent pain when breastfeeding report experiencing aversion, women who have experienced previous sexual abuse report experiencing aversion, women who are 'touched out' and who feel severely sleep deprived report experiencing aversion and women are stressed about their education, or starting back at their job while maintaining their breastfeeding relationship, report experiencing aversion. Women with nurslings who have severe allergies and cannot simply switch to formula or eat regular foodstuffs experience aversion. In each of these scenarios it takes only a little common sense to see why feelings of anger, agitation, irritability and thoughts of wanting to stop breastfeeding may arise. For example, it is very clear why mothers who have been victims of sexual abuse can experience aversion. They have been violated and traumatised, emotionally hurt – and the hurt has been to do with their body and bodily autonomy. As the human brain develops with the environment and isn't just genetically programmed, it can be difficult for the brain to completely separate previous situations from current ones, especially if the mother is the type of person who quickly moves from a state of relaxation to a state of fear, and therefore is more sensitive to shifts in negative emotion.* Any situations that echo past trauma, or even the thought process of a memory of past trauma, can be enough to trigger the same reactions of panic and fight or flight, and therefore the same hormones flood

---

* People with anxiety may strategically choose worrying over relaxing. (n.d.). Retrieved 22 October 2019, from ScienceDaily website: www.sciencedaily.com/releases/2019/09/190930114737.htm

your system and you experience the same negative reaction to stress. These hormones literally change your biological state. Some researchers even believe that they change your biology over time, while others think that traumatic events can affect your health and even change your brain.[*] Imagine being stressed and reliving trauma in some way every time you breastfeed, every single day and night, for months, perhaps years on end. It is no wonder that some of these women are vulnerable to aversion, particularly as their nursling gets older.

Night-times are the worst as they feed for comfort a lot and when they have been there a while I get an overwhelming feeling of claustrophobia, queasy, hot and panicky. I literally want to get them off me and throw them to the other side of the bed (I don't of course) but mum guilt kicks in big style. A few deep breaths and I try to relax again – which sometimes works. They are ultra-clingy at the moment during the day too. Not helped by having a cold. But there is no escaping as they are crawling and pulling themselves up so day and night I am one giant climbing frame that just gets clawed and slapped and pinched and bitten. I feel like I am going crazy. I need space. I need not to be touched. But I have nowhere to go, and they need me. Farah, Nairobi

Looking at the bigger picture it is clear that the benefits to nurslings are seldom the only relevant factors in decisions about infant feeding. Your mental wellbeing as a mother, the competing demands on your time, the impact of breastfeeding on your emotional state and the family home are all factors to consider when we think of the 'superiority' of breastfeeding, and why it may not always be best for you as a mother.[**] There's

[*]   Chen, F., Ke, J., Qi, R., Xu, Q., Zhong, Y., Liu, T., … Lu, G. (2018). Increased Inhibition of the Amygdala by the mPFC may Reflect a Resilience Factor in Post-traumatic Stress Disorder: A Resting-State fMRI Granger Causality Analysis. *Frontiers in Psychiatry*, 9.

[**] Why breastfeeding is not always best – for mother or baby. Laura Frances Callahan, Aeon Essays. (n.d.). Retrieved 22 October 2019, from Aeon website: aeon.co/essays/why-breastfeeding-is-not-always-best-for-mother-or-baby

something almost freeing about accepting this. However, it has taken me many years to accept that it may be the case that breastfeeding for as long as I did was probably not the best thing for me to do. And I am not entirely sure that I would have stopped breastfeeding earlier, even if I had realised it, because of the sort of Stockholm syndrome in the breastfeeding relationship being so strong. I blame oxytocin. I had fallen in love with my captor, and did everything to support and protect them. But I wish that I had had more information to decide, I wish I had had the words to describe what was going on with aversion, and known the possible reasons why it was happening to me. That is what this book intends to do, for all its flaws and inevitable inconsistencies. I hope it offers some insight and allows you as a mother to conduct a simple, honest, self-assessment of your situation and your ability to breastfeed. It takes time and energy to identify sources of friction in your everyday life, and not only what is triggering the experience of aversion in you, but also what the underlying causes are, and to make a change. I believe we already have everything we need to do this, that we already have enough within us to start, and that we will find the answers and solutions in the process, because nurture doesn't stop and we will adapt our breastfeeding relationship, even if it needs to come to an end because of aversion. When we have more knowledge we are empowered to change things, and with aversion it is important to be proactive to prevent it from happening, or getting worse. As with many aspects of child-rearing, it is best to implement things gradually, and in turn expect change gradually. If aversion is plaguing your life, start today by making some small changes using the steps in BROMPHALICC as applicable to you and your nursling. The reason there is nothing prescriptive in this book is because your circumstance and situation is highly specific, and so the cause of aversion will likely be specific to you – even though it is rooted in physiology and psychology for all of us.

Research and evidence-based knowledge

We live in an age where we know so much about so much. There are detailed theories, thousands of journals and books, and media programmes on almost every area of our lives – from health to wealth, the living and the abstract world, in art and in literature. Yet, in our daily lives, particularly as mothers, we are still left with so many unanswered questions. After reading up on a topic to be better informed you can be left more confused than when you started! And to add insult to injury, the information we have doesn't seem to have the desired effect. We know so much about healthy eating, but obesity is on the rise. We know that modern lives are full of stress, and how inflammation due to stress is the main cause of depression, yet depression is going to be the second most prevalent disease in the world. Knowing things doesn't translate into knowing *what to do*. We know so much about the science of breastfeeding, the importance of attachment in development, the natural normal behaviours of children... but as mothers we still don't know whether we should swaddle, why a baby doesn't sleep or the reason some incessantly cry. Blaming 'colic' isn't an answer because colic isn't a reason, colic is a set of symptoms, one of which is continuous crying for long periods of time. We have known benefits of breastfeeding, and the risks of introducing formula early, but not how to weigh all the infant feeding options in light of the mental and emotional costs that mothers incur. With aversion we don't know if we should carry on breastfeeding despite hating it and experiencing negative emotions, because we don't know if our nurslings will be harmed if we stop. It certainly seems as though we are harming them if we deny them the comfort and closeness of suckling, the skinship and nurture that they are accustomed to.

The exponential amount of knowledge and research, and its accessibility, arguably makes being a mother a difficult thing to do despite the wealth of information out there – we are always second-guessing ourselves. One reason is because even though there is instant access to so much information, it is often conflicting, and most of it is well presented so you feel you ought to take the advice, only to find a contradictory position that seems just as valid. Turning to the internet, academic books, and even family and friends to figure out what to do isn't always the best strategy either, because taking research findings and trying to implement them in a complex family life will probably not work unless you know everything about the research and your situation, with an outsider's objective perspective. Evidence-based research is so important in our modern-day decision-making, as educated women, but without proper interpretation it can add false expectations to mothers' lives. Have you heard of the research that shows that breastfeeding mothers get more sleep than mothers who formula feed? Do you tell other women about it? I wouldn't, unless in direct response to someone who claims formula-feeding mothers get more sleep because their babies' tummies are filled with formula milk. This is not because it is untrue, but because of *how much* more sleep the study says breastfeeding mothers get. It's half an hour. Half an hour!* The study is useful to prove a point. It is not useful for a mother on the brink of despair due to sleep deprivation. And it is not useful for breastfeeding mothers with aversion.

Another example is that many people now know about the research that shows that breastfeeding is protective against depression, but the key to the truth of this statement is that it is protective only when *breastfeeding is going well.* This doesn't much help us minority breastfeeding mothers with aversion who appear to be outliers. As a researcher, and when I read clinical trial protocols for my research ethics committee, I often see variables in research having to be reduced to the bare minimum in order for a topic to be researched. I've always wondered how this affected the results in each study. Even if we are researching a simple thing, or giving research

---

*   Doan, T., Gay, C. L., Kennedy, H. P., Newman, J., & Lee, K. A. (2014). Nighttime breastfeeding behavior is associated with more nocturnal sleep among first-time mothers at one month postpartum. *Journal of Clinical Sleep Medicine: JCSM: Official Publication of the American Academy of Sleep Medicine, 10*(3), 313–319. *Journal of Clinical Sleep Medicine: JCSM: Official Publication of the American Academy of Sleep Medicine, 10*(3), 313–319.

participants a simple question to answer, it would be naive to think they were not thinking of anything else except that task or that question. They are probably wondering if they are correctly answering the question, or wanting another box to tick because it does not accurately reflect their response. Holt describes this well when he says 'there is another very profoundly mistaken assumption in all research: with what we can learn about people in a very limited, unusual, and often very anxious situation we can make reliable judgements about what they do in the very different and more usual situations'.* The things people say and how they behave when they are research participants is different from normal everyday life for them.

No amount of statistics can give us the kind of understanding we need as breastfeeding mothers. If we found out that from 1,000 breastfeeding journeys, 400 women have challenges, from which half (or 200) experienced aversion to varying degrees, we would have a 20 percent statistic or a ratio of two from every ten with symptoms of aversion. But that doesn't tell me anything important about aversion, the difficulties of bodily autonomy and consent, when aversion can start and why, or the tension and conflict that is experienced. Without a more detailed understanding, reference to the wider picture and the lived experience of women who were almost always sovereign over their bodies before motherhood, I think research about breastfeeding taken out of context can add a level of *cognitive dissonance* in us. This is a description of the psychological stress or mental discomfort you can feel when you hold contradictory beliefs and values, which is often triggered when the ideas you hold clash with new evidence presented to you. When it comes to studies in breastfeeding and parenting, we have to ask ourselves when reading research headlines and statements, how does this apply to me as a breastfeeding mother in the real world, in my particular circumstances? What can I learn from this study, or this recommendation in my *personal situation*?

---

* Holt, J. (1995). *How Children Fail* (Rev. Ed edition). Reading, Mass: DaCapo Press, p9.

Mothers who are at their wits' end, who have a baby screaming, or a toddler who wakes 15 times at night, will try to do something about it by researching what can help. Sleep and sleep interventions are one of the most common areas parents find stressful and so they are keen to improve their nurslings sleep, spending a great deal of time and energy to manipulate the sleep environment and 'train' their nursling. But if we knew before all intervention that co-parenting is an independent variable for child sleep, we would focus on our relationship with our partner, and try to cooperate by sharing the load in order to get our nursling to have better sleep and fewer wakes. Imagine reading the 1,001 things you have to try to get your child to sleep, spending hundreds on sleep products from white noise machines to lavender diffusers to weighted blankets, when all the while your child was waking because you argue with your partner and both of you are stressed!

My point is, even if some research is irrefutably correct, even if breastmilk is amazing, even if the most important stage of childhood development is the formative years – what does it matter to us, if the research doesn't include the reality of life as a mother in the 21st century? We talk about 'biological norms' as if they were the gold standard of how to act and how to behave, without taking into account societal changes and cultural changes. We have moved away from many biological norms. No wonder there is some cognitive dissonance, disconnect, and daily struggle for mothers who think they are doing it all as they are 'supposed to', to provide the best for their nurslings. We may have internalised that breastfeeding and responsive parenting is best for our nurslings, but we haven't taken into account that culture can override this and make biological norms difficult or even obsolete.* With the rise in formula use worldwide, breastfeeding is not needed for a nursling to survive. And mothers can feel this in the way that the job of mothering and the job of breastfeeding are continually undermined in society. The Industrial Revolution wasn't that long ago, and factory life, supply and demand

---

* Dettwyler, K.A. (1995). Sexuality and Breastfeeding. *Journal of Human Lactation*, 11(4), 263–263.

of goods, working 9–5 and a change in societal structure came with it. Arguably, as women in society, we are still in the reactive throes of dealing with the artificial construct of time being forced onto our rhythmic, natural, biologically normal way of living as mothers and babies. It has, in many ways, completely replaced it. Biological clocks are no longer what we follow, nor are they protected or promoted. How can we be the best mothers we can be when we are still fighting incorrect advice about feeding little tiny humans 'every three or four hours', and are still faced with the prevalent, but false, idea that babies and children can sleep for 12 hours straight at night? Mothering can be very hard for some, and it is not uncommon to feel like you are drowning. The tensions and conflicts between the biological norms of pre-modernity, and the juxtaposed positions promoted in life in modernity certainly affect us as breastfeeding mothers today. By giving us false expectations, by overwhelming us with the unreachable pedestal of perfection as a mother and by stealing our time and attention so that little is left to care for our nurslings and for ourselves.[*]

The cost of love, and the expression of survival

Does it cost us to love? It certainly costs us as caregivers to care. If this is considered synonymous with love and loving your offspring, you could say that it does 'cost' us a great deal to love. Endorphins make possible the experience of love, and the attachment of parent and child. They also are our own natural painkillers, helping us reduce feelings of pain and to deal with stress. Other hormones like dopamine and oxytocin also interact this way. Why do mothers with aversion seem to have a temporary fault with these hormones? Why do mothers with aversion seem to have a suppression of oxytocin, or upregulation of the stress response when oxytocin is released? Dopamine is released when we experience pleasure,

---

[*]   See Intensive Mothering in the Hays, S. (1998). *The Cultural Contradictions of Motherhood*. Yale University Press.

so why don't some women get this hit of dopamine when breastfeeding? All the good parts of how motherly love is meant to be experienced seem to be missing when we consider the phenomenon of aversion, its causes and triggers. I wonder if caregiver burnout happens in mothers with aversion, with a change in attitude from positive and caring to negative and more distant: fatigue of being compassionate at one's own cost. Without physical support from other people, in person, to help mothers out, without the guidance of people who actually know what they are talking about, and without the close communities seen in older generations or tribal living that would share the load of responsibility, mothers simply cannot cope. Healthcare professionals get compassion fatigue, as caring is recognised as a draining role. If they do, why wouldn't mothers? The term compassion fatigue was first used to describe burnout, but interestingly it is now understood by many to be a secondary traumatic stress disorder from looking after patients who are in pain or discomfort.[*] Things are never quite as they seem in research. Humans are always affected in more than one way, on more than one level.

Aside from mentioning a mother's love earlier in this book, I have not brought it up again because I have tried to write at length about birth interventions, stress and any number of combinations of biological, psychological and social aspects that can inhibit our ability to mother. This means they also inhibit learning to love, giving love, and nurturing love. As Penny Van Esterik would contend, they would all compromise our ability as mothers to do the 'dance of nurture', because dancing is really all about love.[**] Love, with help from the positive aspects of oxytocin, can help us bear the pain of motherhood, the challenges, the sleep interruptions and the

---

[*]   Coetzee, S.K., & Klopper, H.C. (2010). Compassion fatigue within nursing practice: A concept analysis. *Nursing & Health Sciences*, *12*(2), 235–243.

[**] See Van Esterik, P. (2017). *The dance of nurture: Negotiating infant feeding*. New York : Berghahn Books, where she conceptualising breastfeeding as nurture, describing the dance of nurture as distinct from industrialised patterns of infant feeding and the corresponding words used to describe the latter (supply and demand, timed feeds etc).

sacrifices we personally make. Without it we can quickly move into low moods and depression. But love doesn't just magically appear for many mothers – despite the expectation that it will and therefore the notion that it ought. Love for some has to be worked on, especially if the start of the relationship with your nursling was rocky.

Working on building love is key to helping alleviate aversion for many reasons, and also to help weaning from the breast, to replace the closeness and bond that breastfeeding has created. A mother working on loving her new self, despite the loss of her original self, can also help move away from the guilt and shame. Part of experiencing negative emotions like guilt and shame is self-loathing – which you cannot have when you love yourself. When we consider love, or being in love, as a breastfeeding mother, it could mean the difference between you willingly submitting to being held prisoner (of sorts) by your nursling, and feeling constricted and constrained against your will. Don't get me wrong: by mentioning love I am not placing a judgement on mothers who struggle to love. I have often wondered if the ability to love, or the lack of it, is wholly down to us, or if it is a combination of things that may have happened before, during or after becoming a mother. In short, it can take more work to love for some mothers.

Modernity has put mothers under a new level of pressure. How could this not affect our breastfeeding relationships? I see a direct correlation. Even if you are unable to do more and be more, our 21st-century environment encourages us to find personal fulfilment outside of mothering. This subconsciously undermines what we do, and makes the task of mothering harder.

Do you have a sense of purpose, even a sense of achievement? Do you have feelings of happiness, serenity, or control in your life – even temporarily? If not, then maybe aversion when breastfeeding isn't the actual problem, but a sign that these qualities are missing from your life. I am not suggesting that you should, or even can have them in your life – I am just asking you to ask yourself if they are absent, and why. I can think of one good reason why they may be absent. If you look at the basic requirements for taking care of a baby or toddler, Robin Grille suggests that there needs to be at least four or up to eight caregivers to one child.* You can be interrupted every two minutes when they are awake, because they always need something. The requests for interaction from some nurslings can be incredibly high, but even without these mothers still have to keep their children from harming themselves, which can mean constant monitoring. Isn't this reason enough to experience aversion, when the demands related to caregiving fall only on you? If we live in such a way that help and support is in great abundance, it is easy to be nurturing because the load is shared. If we live in such a way that a lot of the burden is on us, we may find nurturing more challenging.

Not only is caregiving challenging mentally, but it is also challenging physically: many of the demands of an infant necessitate body contact, day and night without proper rest. Rest comes in many forms: not just sleep, but also having time away, and solitude to recharge, the permission to not be helpful or to do things for your family, a break from responsibility. If we were truly to rest we would need to be totally unproductive, we would need to have stillness to decompress and a safe space to have alone time at home, none of which mothers get consistently.

Our systems of education and work do not fit well into mothering in the early intensive years of childcare, and the homemaker is not respected in modern life. Centuries of idealising mothering and a mother's role have created phantasms of what love as a mother entails, and how breastfeeding ought to be experienced, but for many they are just not true. Breastfeeding is painful and boring and frustrating, and although you do not have to like breastfeeding to do it, you do have to be committed to be able to do it through challenging phases of breastfeeding and to meet the needs of your nursling(s). Add to this the pressures of modern-day life that can inflate inside us over time – like a balloon with air being pumped in – too much pressure and it will pop, and all

---

* Grille, R. (2013). *Parenting for a Peaceful World* (Second Edition edition). New South Wales, Australia: Vox Cordis Press.

the air will come rushing out. These are our paroxysms of rage when we get aversion.

Controlling ourselves is just as hard as being controlled. Refraining from acting on negative emotions, and continuing to be responsive when everything inside you is screaming to run away, takes great will: a sincere intention and strong resolve to continue to breastfeed, to continue to *mother through breastfeeding.* The battle is real with aversion, which was once described to me as similar to a 'wave of nausea: something you didn't know was coming, but once it hit you, you damn well knew it was there'. Having aversion tests your intention, your resolve to breastfeed, and your power of self-control as a person. Having a sense of autonomy over your body as a free agent – a sense of being able to do or not do an action as you wish – is often compromised as a mother. This is important because agency is demonstrated by making choices, but with aversion as a breastfeeding mother, you cannot simply decide what happens to your own body there and then. And many mothers find their internal control and self-governance override what they want or need to do, in order to keep giving nurslings 'their' milk, from your body. Recognising this predicament is something I wanted this book to do, because it is not stated anywhere else, and so it is as if this difficulty doesn't exist.

Many of us know, either experientially, or from well-known research in attachment parenting, that responsiveness increases attachment and emotional intelligence, and that there is a clear link between empathy and breastfeeding. We know that we cannot just turn off responsive care, day or night: we do not ignore the cries and the needs of our nurslings.[*] Many of us do not want to give non-human milk in a bottle, or allow someone else to feed our young, for many, many reasons – and we should not have to justify this. Yet the insistence that some women can continue to give and give through responsive caregiving, through responsive breastfeeding, and find fulfilment at home with a nursling is a cruel fantasy that

---

[*] Ainsworth, M. S., & Bowlby, J. (1991). An ethological approach to personality development. *American Psychologist*, 46(4), 333–341.

exacerbates aversion for them. If mothers are drowning in motherhood, their survival mode will kick in, and when stuck in the difficult situation of being primary caregivers with no respite, stress reactivity becomes a pattern in their lives.

Adding another layer of complexity into aversion, we know this stress is contagious: with mirror neurons and our social nervous system offline, aversion affects our nurslings. Perhaps not when aversion strikes sporadically, but certainly when it becomes chronic or experienced for a longer period of time. Our relationship with our nurslings becomes compromised, and this can be upsetting and an additional emotional burden. This is not what is meant to happen, you tell yourself. This is not the kind of mother I am. I agree, and I would say you are not that mother, you are just responding to an intolerable situation.

Is this the book that will answer all the questions we have about aversion? Not at all, and I hope no one would ever claim that a piece of work or research could do so: research will always change and expand our understanding. Paradigm shifts in any field will mean what we once thought was true becomes untrue and is supplanted by a new theory, a new way of understanding a problem or reality. For example, the foremilk and hindmilk theory has recently been retired, after being promoted for many years, because it is now understood to be incorrect. Theories are just that, theories and not facts. They are just a way of understanding something. One theory won't ever apply to everything or everyone, and from what I can see, we mothers with aversion have to contend with the difficulties of being the outliers in theory and research. The predominant view that breastfeeding is good and therefore what is best for mother and nursling doesn't really apply to us. We are the ones that struggle with breastfeeding, often until the bitter end, the ones with super-sensitive nipples, the ones with a baby that sleeps on the lower end of the bell curve (ie, that does not sleep), the ones dealing with cow's milk protein allergy and other allergies, or tri-feeding with formula and pumping as well as breastfeeding. We are mothers that want it all – to be the perfect happily in love breastfeeding mother

– but have no way of getting there and so feel ever more stuck. We are the ones whose efforts at responsiveness through breastfeeding no longer increase attachment, and for whom skinship in its literal sense is compromised.

We mothers tend to put our nurslings first. When thinking about breastfeeding mothers we have to assume there are elements of self-preservation when we try to address aversion, because we all know the self-sacrifice narrative of mothers. Of course a certain amount of self-sacrifice is necessary, because without us our nurslings would not survive, but do we not have some biological mechanisms in place to ensure our own survival? A way to come back from the madness of 'giving your all'? Aversion, perhaps? There is, in this way, a positive aspect to the struggle with the emotions that can arise if you experience aversion. Mothers can and do use the experience of aversion and the 'negative' feelings as a source of energy to shift a dynamic, as a catalyst for change and transformation: a natural first step in the body speaking to you to instigate the process of weaning (and weaning is a *process*, not a singular event of breastfeeding cessation).

The fact that aversion can be an important signal for change is a key message of this book, along with my observational analysis that the experience of aversion is actually a key medical indicator, or a *sign*, of other underlying issues that need to be addressed. The self-reported symptoms of aversion, when taken in context with a mother's previous medical and personal history, can and do point to clear reasons why she may be experiencing aversion. And on a simpler, less medical level, whether aversion is the biological trigger for older nurslings to start weaning, or because of the stress response triggered, or simply because a mother is unsupported and feels unhappy, aversion is an indication to change something. That doesn't necessarily mean physically, because as a biopsychosocial phenomenon much of aversion can be in our own minds. Being stuck breastfeeding and unable to distract yourself from your current situation means you can't get away from your own mind, your own thoughts. As young independent women before motherhood we used to go out, and move away from things we didn't like by throwing ourselves into work or socialising to escape from the 'self'. As mothers we can no longer do that. And while it can be easy to blame everyone and the world for our mood and our actions, there is an argument that suggests that what comes out is what we are all holding inside, and there is no better situation than the constraints of breastfeeding nurslings to bring out all of that anger, all of that grief. A good way to illustrate this is to look at what happens when you are holding a cup of tea and someone walks past and accidentally bumps into you, spilling the tea all over the floor and yourself. Why did the tea spill? One reason is clear: someone bumped into you. But there is another way to look at it, another valid reason: you spilled the tea because there was tea in the cup. Whatever was in the cup would have spilled out. The idea here is that what is inside you will spill out when life hits you. Is there joy, happiness, and peace in you, or anger, resentment and frustration? And while I think you cannot completely choose to have the former, there is some level of choice we have, and work we can do to fill our cups with kindness, gentleness and love, so that what spills over to our nurslings is the same as what is inside us. However, I don't think it is possible to do this until we understand our triggers for aversion, or deal with its real cause, whether biological, psychological or social. And sometimes it isn't possible for mothers to do it without weaning.

Positive aspects of aversion

Aversion is a chance to recognise that something needs to shift; that something needs healing; that something isn't quite right in feeding and interacting with your nursling, or in your life. Reframing the experience of aversion can help you use it as a growth experience. Some mothers maintain that not only breastfeeding, but also breastfeeding aversion, defines them as a mother. Aversion has taught them that their will and their determination can override their minds and bodies. It is an opportunity to learn how *not* to react, what their personal limits are as mothers, and that sometimes, putting themselves first is best for everyone.

> *In a way I'm even a little bit grateful for aversion for it taught me that I can't do it all on my own, that I do need others, as well as that I need to look after myself and listen to my own body. Self-care when going through aversion was what made mine better.* Bianca, Geneva

Listening to the inner voice that is screaming out when aversion manifests is not a bad thing. Self-sacrifice is something we get used to when we become mothers, so that our nurslings survive and then thrive, but letting it continue as they get older and you cannot cope can turn this self-sacrifice into an emergency situation. As attachment parents who nurture and have created a special skinship, this *putting themselves first* becomes very difficult. But in an emergency situation, it is standard operating procedure to put yourself first, just as with oxygen masks on airplanes. Aversion is a nudge that if not heeded, can end up forcing you to make a change. Often, if making reductions or changes to the breastfeeding relationship doesn't work, especially for older nurslings, it is the difficulty in accepting weaning that prevents us from moving forward. We have to remind ourselves that there is a strong case for aversion being normal in the natural world, along with maternal aggression and refusal of the breast. In the animal world, there are many examples of maternal mammalian aggression toward suckling infants, such as like lionesses hitting clambering cubs and sows (female pigs) rolling over and crushing suckling piglets to death.* What if, for some mothers, child-led weaning wasn't the right thing to do? What if some of us are meant to wean our nurslings when they are one or two years old? If you are experiencing aversion with an older nursling, it doesn't go away when you have taken

---

* Johnson, A. K., Morrow, J. L., Dailey, J. W., & McGlone, J. J. (2007). Pre-weaning mortality in loose-housed lactating sows: Behavioral and performance differences between sows who crush or do not crush piglets. *Applied Animal Behaviour Science*, *105*(1–3), 59–74. doi. org/10.1016/j.applanim.2006.06.001

the steps using BROMPHALICC, or even gets worse, it would be worth considering stopping breastfeeding, as this is literally what aversion is telling you to do.

For other mothers, as aversion is an indicator of something else going on, it is worth considering the woman behind aversion. When I was a baby I contracted polio from a vaccination. I had partial paralysis of my right leg and a little bit of scoliosis in my back. Other than a whole bunch of operations and spending half of my life in hospital, having polio didn't really affect me physically. I also never felt 'disabled' having it. I used to bike for miles at night to see friends, go out to dance for hours (with an orthotic brace), and I even ran a badminton club when I was working for the NHS. A few years ago, however, I started to get very tired if I had had a busy day. I would have to regroup my body and mind by doing nothing, and I had to recuperate by sleeping a lot. If I didn't sleep enough, it would be more painful for me to walk, everything seemed harder and I would spend the day fighting to get through it until I could sleep. There were times when I could sleep 12 hours a night and I would still have to lie down to rest during the day. If I made more than one plan in a day I would get terrible shooting pains in my leg, all day forehead headaches and persistent eye strain. Looking back, my body was very clearly saying 'no, stop'. My body was stopping me from carrying on. Fast-forward eight years and I have been diagnosed with post-polio syndrome: neuropathic pain, relentless fatigue, new muscle weakness and persistent falls. It was a difficult time and I often felt frustrated that I wasn't understood and had no answers for my symptoms, until I became involved in a polio community and at once felt like I belonged. My pain, my struggles – which seemed invisible to others – were instantly understood and I no longer needed to explain myself. My small achievements in life with managing polio were celebrated. I had a funny sense of pride – polio pride, if you will. This is the same kind of pride I feel when I am around people who understand breastfeeding, the importance of breastfeeding and the difficulties of breastfeeding through aversion. We breastfeeding mothers are not understood by most of society, including healthcare professionals, and that makes our struggles invisible too. Breastfeeding pride – and breastfeeding through aversion – is a defining part of the journey of motherhood for some mothers. We haven't been around mothers who are mothering their entire lives; those days are gone now with planned parenthood and feminist waves, but when we are in a mothering community where we feel comfortable to say we are breastfeeding, bed-sharing and even experiencing aversion, we can start to feel proud. We can have a true sense of accomplishment among those who understand what doing these things *cost* us. These mothers understand our experiences – both good and bad – and offer great insights without trying to fix the situation or change the way in which we mother. Intuitively, they respect and honour both skinship and nurture, in their understanding of what breastfeeding is in reality. They don't see our breastfeeding relationship with our nurslings as a problem, nor the fact we are stuck mothering as a tragedy or something to be ashamed of. They appreciate how much it sucks when a partner won't get up and take the baby in the morning because they have been attached to you all night, allowing you to vent and complain about how much you hate breastfeeding. They appreciate how much it sucks when aversion strikes, ruining everything.

Not everyone understands breastfeeding pride, which is apparent when a mother stops breastfeeding and people nearly always repeat the same remarks: 'You can go out without the baby'. 'You are free at night now'. 'You can get your body back'. I can't say hearing these things didn't get to me when I stopped, even though they are partly true. It's just that these comments diminish the lives of breastfeeding mothers, especially those with aversion. Even if we are suffering, we do not necessarily want to be cured by stopping breastfeeding – despite all that heartache it can bring. We want to be supported to breastfeed, we desperately want to enjoy it, we want to be the mother we dreamed we would be, with limitless patience and limitless responsiveness: we want to cherish time with our nurslings as a mother, and enjoy breastfeeding, but we can't. Aversion is crushing.

Wouk and colleagues showed that there was a relationship between maternal positive emotions during feeding and breastfeeding outcomes – that women fed for longer durations.* You would think that maternal negative emotions would then lead to women feeding for shorter durations, but for many women with aversion the relationship to breastfeeding outcomes is that women *struggle when feeding*. We can see this in the experience of so many mothers, the emotional turmoil of struggling with managing the breastfeeding relationship and everything that is compromised when aversion strikes. In breastfeeding communities that understand and accept aversion we see mothers being able to accept who they are and what they are going through. They have had horrible and soul-destroying experiences, as well as beautiful and rich experiences, not in spite of, but because of being a breastfeeding mother with aversion. In the end, they have come to understand that as mothers they will love, and they will hate. They will love, and they will grieve. And breastfeeding is just one step in the journey of motherhood; aversion is just one point on the timeline and perceived failures do not define who you are as a mother overall. The heartache of knowing your firstborn will take second place when you fall pregnant, the guilt you feel when you cannot carry on breastfeeding until they want to wean, the shame you feel at failing because you are not constantly responding as a happy mother. These are early points in a long timeline: you will have plenty of opportunities to become the mother you always wanted to be, the mother you know you can be. When you are in the emotional sleep-deprived storm, it can seem you have failed at it all. You haven't. Just because you could not cope as a mother of younger nurslings does not mean you cannot be a caring, supportive mother to your child when they are struggling at school, or as a young adult who is going through relationship troubles or a life crisis. There are plenty of opportunities to be the mother you always wanted to be as your nursling grows,

---

* Positive Emotions During Infant Feeding and Breastfeeding Outcomes. PubMed—NCBI. (n.d.). Retrieved 11 October 2019, from www.ncbi. nlm.nih.gov/pubmed/31059653

and there will be many other times as a mother when you will excel at being present, responsive and caring into adulthood. There is time to heal, there is time to 'get it right' outside of breastfeeding, and the bonds of skinship will continue and grow to be stronger even if aversion has temporarily compromised them. While it may be hard to see if you are in the thick of it, looking at mothering across a whole lifetime, you can see that the first few years are but a tiny fraction of your child's entire life, and their relationship with you is yet to fully develop. Interpersonal touch is an important part of all relationships, and as your nurslings grow older you can have more contact in ways that will promote better relationships and improve your individual wellbeing. Even hugging will start to be associated with a positive effect and reduced conflict all round as the negative emotions triggered by touch and breastfeeding no longer arise. So you will hug, and you will love, and they will hug and you will love it, and in the end, all shall be well.

Further Resources

There are many breastfeeding/nursing aversion support groups on Facebook. The one I manage is called *Aversion Sucks – Peer to Peer Breastfeeding Support*.

Breastfeeding Older Babies and Beyond is also a great breastfeeding support group on Facebook too, for information and solidarity when it's tough with older nurslings.

The Cleavage Club (USA), *UK Breastfeeding and Parenting Support* and *Breastfeeding Yummy Mummies* (UK) are wonderful for breastfeeding support in the early months – with infant feeding trained admin from peer supporters to IBCLCs.

It is worth mentioning that it can be hard to be a part of more traditional breastfeeding support groups if a mother suffers severe aversion because intense negative emotions and/or weaning are not often spoken about in these groups, and the remit of the groups is to support and encourage breastfeeding. However, joining in conjunction with an aversion support group can be helpful for evidenced-based information, and if mothers wish to continue breastfeeding. For sleep *The Beyond Sleep Training Project* and *Biologically Normal Infant and Toddler Sleep* Facebook groups are invaluable and evidenced-based.

Blogs and articles for further reading:

La Leche League: www.laleche.org.uk/dont-enjoy-breastfeeding

Milk and Motherhood: www.milkandmotherhood.com/2017/01/nursing-aversion-or-wanting-to-scream

Peggy O'Mara: www.peggyomara.com/2019/09/23/breastfeeding-aversion-and-agitation

Lycra Widow: www.lycrawidow.com/2016/07/08/on-the-edge-get-off-me

Mother Love: www.motherlove.com/blogs/all/negative-emotions-while-breastfeeding

The Motherload: www.the-motherload.co.uk/8-tips-for-managing-breastfeeding-aversion

The Pulse: blog.pregistry.com/breastfeeding-agitation-aversion

Sarah Ockwell-Smith: www.sarahockwell-smith.com

BASIS (Evidenced-based Sleep Information): www.basisonline.org.uk

Index